HOMEOPATHY

HOMEOPATHY
HARNESSING NATURE'S PHARMACY

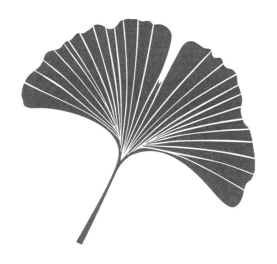

EMMA VAN HINSBERGH

SIRIUS

All illustrations courtesy of Shutterstock

SIRIUS

This edition published in 2024 by Sirius Publishing, a division of
Arcturus Publishing Limited,
26/27 Bickels Yard, 151–153 Bermondsey Street,
London SE1 3HA

ISBN: 978-1-3988-4465-0
AD011466UK

Printed in China

CONTENTS

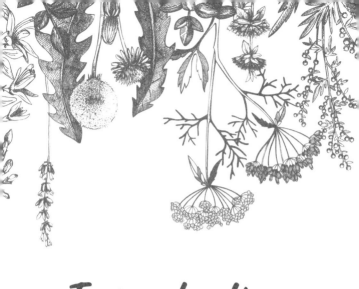

Introduction

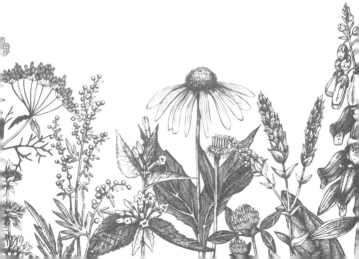

Within the realm of complementary medicine, one particular healing modality has intrigued and captivated millions around the world for centuries: homeopathy. Developed over 200 years ago by the German physician Samuel Hahnemann, homeopathy is a gentle system of medicine based on the principle of 'like cures like.'

This subtle yet powerful method of healing uses minute doses of naturally occurring substances extracted from plants and minerals to stimulate the body's vital force or inherent healing energy to restore balance and well-being.

While it is often grouped together with other natural and integrative therapies such as herbal medicine, flower essences or aromatherapy, homeopathy has its own unique set of rules and protocols which have been rigorously honed over the centuries. With its own distinct medicines, production methods, training programmes, professional organisations and certification standards, it really is in a class of its own.

What's more, because the remedies are administered in such miniscule amounts, they can usually be used alongside conventional medical treatment, under the guidance of a professional, so homeopathy really is a complementary therapy.

Holistic harmony

The central philosophy of homeopathy is based on the belief that your body has an innate ability to heal itself, and that symptoms of illness are your body's way of trying to restore balance.

A homeopath's goal is to stimulate your natural healing process by prescribing holistic remedies that match your symptoms, personality, and overall constitution.

Encompassing a truly holistic approach to health, homeopathy acknowledges the important connection between mind, body and spirit and

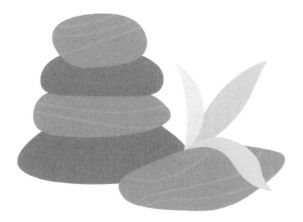

addresses the root cause of the issue rather than focusing solely on alleviating symptoms, as tends to be the case in conventional medicine. By taking into consideration your unique physical, emotional, and mental characteristics, homeopathy aims to stimulate your body's vital force, and bring you back to health and equilibrium.

What's more, because it's such a safe and gentle healing mode, you can use it to treat many minor health niggles at home. Why not try arnica to soothe knocks and bruises, apis mel for insect stings or agnus castus to improve your memory? There's a whole treasure trove of subtle yet incredibly effective remedies out there to help you, your family and even your pets.

By using this book as a handy tool to delve more deeply into this fascinating healing system, you can learn how to improve your mind, body and soul. From getting a better night's sleep to boosting your immune system, homeopathy can set you on the road to a healthier, happier life.

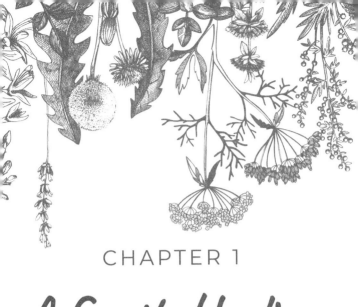

CHAPTER 1

A Gentle Healing Tradition

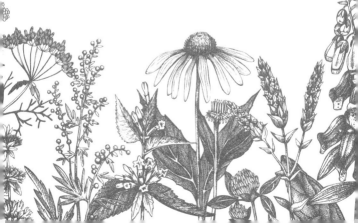

THE HISTORY OF HOMEOPATHY

While the basic principle of homeopathy was used by the ancient Greeks (the word homeopathy was derived from the word 'homoios' meaning 'at one with' or 'the same as'), modern homeopathy as we know it was developed in the late 18th century by a visionary German physician called Samuel Hahnemann. Known as the 'Father of Homeopathy', he became dissatisfied with the harsh and not particularly effective medical practices of his time, which included bloodletting,

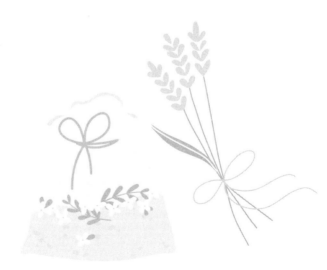

purging and the use of toxic substances, and sought to find an alternative approach to these somewhat brutal treatments.

While translating a medical treatise by a Scottish physician called William Cullen, which described use of the poisonous cinchona bark (quinine) to treat malaria, he made a key discovery: Experimenting on himself, he discovered that taking the potent raw bark induced fever, chills and joint pain—symptoms similar to those of the disease itself. This led him to develop the homeopathic principle of similarity or 'similia similibus curentur', which means 'let like be treated by like'.

According to this principle, Hahnemann postulated that a substance which caused symptoms in a healthy person could be used in a highly diluted form to treat similar symptoms in a sick person. He tested this theory by conducting experiments on himself and his remarkably accommodating colleagues, known as 'provings', in which they, somewhat bravely, ingested small doses of various substances over a long period and recorded the symptoms they experienced.

Through this and other provings, Hahnemann later compiled a *materia medica*—a collection of remedies and their associated symptoms. Sourced from natural substances such as plants, minerals, and animal products, all the remedies were highly diluted to minimize any potential side effects. This was done through a process he developed of dilution and potentization, which involves a substance being repeatedly diluted and succussed (shaken vigorously) to enhance its therapeutic properties while minimising any toxic effects.

Global healing

In 1810, Hahnemann published his seminal work, *Organon of the Rational Art of Healing*, which outlined the fundamental principles and concepts of homeopathy and became the cornerstone of homeopathic philosophy and practice.

His pioneering work and the principles of homeopathy gained popularity in Europe and eventually spread to other parts of the world, and it became increasingly prevalent in the 19th century and early 20th century, when many renowned homeopathic institutes and schools were established. These included the Hahnemann Medical College in 1835 in Philadelphia, Pennsylvania and the Royal London Homeopathic Hospital in 1849 in London, England.

Famous figures took to it enthusiastically too. Queen Victoria of the United Kingdom reportedly had her own personal homeopath, Dr Frederick Quin, while the revered Indian leader, Mahatma Gandhi, used homeopathy for both acute and chronic conditions.

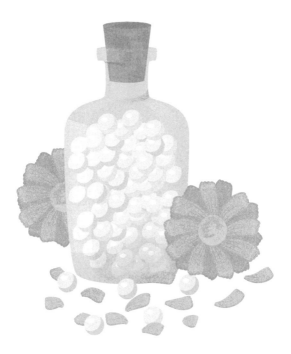

HOMEOPATHY TODAY

While the popularity of homeopathy faced challenges from the rise of conventional medicine and the increasing demand for scientific evidence in the 20th century, it has proved effective for millions of people worldwide. Medical journals have published numerous positive reports of the results of scientific research into homeopathy, and it continues to be practiced by dedicated practitioners and has gained a renewed interest in recent years.

Today, homeopathy remains a popular form of complementary medicine around the world and its principles and remedies are widely used by people seeking a more holistic and individualised approach to health and well-being.

What's more, the research is out there to back it up. A meta-analysis published in *The Lancet* examined 186 studies and found a significant effect of homeopathy beyond placebo. Similarly, a review published in the *British Journal of Clinical Pharmacology* analysed 104 studies and concluded that there is evidence that homeopathy has therapeutic effects. The Homeopathy Research Institute is an excellent source of information if you'd like to look into this further.

Global health

Today, homeopathy is recognised as one of the main complementary and integrative medicine modalities and is practiced by trained homeopaths and healthcare professionals across the globe, from Argentina to Mexico and Switzerland to Spain.

A Global TGI Survey conducted by Kantar Media found that in India, where homeopathy is integrated into the public healthcare system, it is used by 59 per cent of the population, while research conducted by the European Commission found that 29 per cent of Europeans are fans.

Germany also has a long-standing tradition of holistic healing, and it is home to several renowned research institutions, and homeopathy is well-integrated into the healthcare system. Meanwhile, in France, it is practiced by both medical doctors and non-medical practitioners, and some health insurance plans cover homeopathic consultations. In the United Kingdom, homeopathy has a huge following and while it is not integrated into the National Health Service (NHS), some doctors and hospitals offer homeopathic treatments.

The principles of homeopathy

Classical homeopathy is based on three fundamental principles:

1. The law of similars

This is the principle of 'like cures like', which means that a substance that can cause symptoms in a healthy person can also cure similar symptoms in a sick person when it is diluted and prepared in a special way. For example, if a person has a fever and chills, a homeopathic remedy made from a substance that can cause fever and chills in a healthy person, such as belladonna, may be prescribed.

2. The minimum dose

Homeopathic remedies are highly diluted to minimise any potential side effects. This is based on the principle that the more diluted a substance is, the more potent its healing properties become. In fact, many homeopathic remedies are so dilute that they contain little or no measurable amount of the original substance.

3. Individualization

Remedies are always prescribed individually (one remedy at a time) by the study of the whole person. This individualized approach is believed to be more effective than a one-size-fits-all approach. Hahnemann insisted that if the right remedy is selected, then that will work for the person on every level.

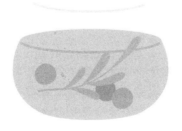

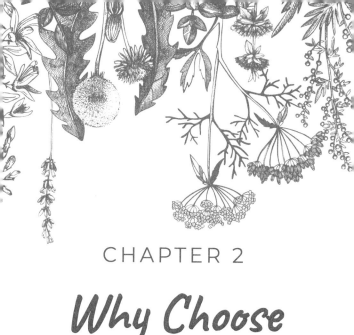

CHAPTER 2

Why Choose Homeopathy?

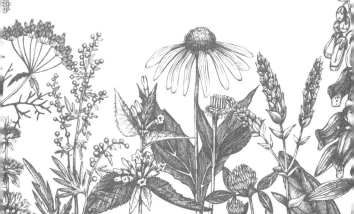

While conventional medicine should be your first port of call for many illnesses and conditions, sometimes a more natural and holistic approach to healthcare can work wonders. As homeopathic remedies are made from such highly diluted substances, they are safe for most people, including babies and children. They are non-toxic and do not typically cause side effects or drug interactions.

Homeopathy aims to treat the person as a whole, taking their physical, mental, and emotional aspects into consideration. More importantly, it recognises the interconnectedness of symptoms and seeks to get to the root of the problems rather than merely suppressing symptoms, as is the case in a lot of conventional treatments.

Homeopathy is often sought for chronic conditions, where conventional medicine might not help in providing long-term relief. It aims to stimulate the body's natural healing abilities, addressing the root cause of the imbalance and promoting overall well-being.

USE WITH OTHER MEDICINES

Homeopathy can be used in conjunction with conventional medicine quite safely and effectively. In fact, many people choose to integrate homeopathic remedies into their overall healthcare approach to complement conventional treatments.

Homeopathy is considered a form of complementary and alternative medicine (CAM), and while it is not a replacement for conventional medicine, especially in cases of life-threatening conditions, it can be used as a complementary approach to conventional treatments, aiding in symptom relief, reducing side effects, and promoting overall well-being.

By working with a qualified homeopath and informing your healthcare provider about your use of homeopathic remedies, you can ensure that your treatments are coordinated and comprehensive. This allows for a more holistic approach to your healthcare, addressing both the symptoms and underlying imbalances.

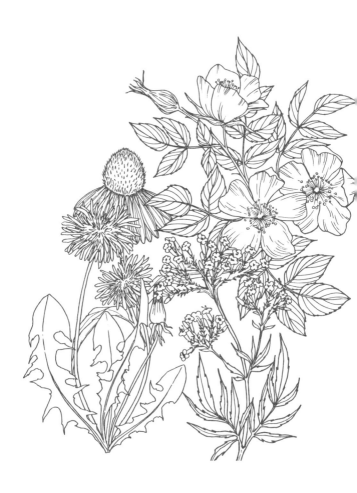

However, it's crucial to consult with healthcare professionals trained in both conventional medicine and homeopathy to ensure proper evaluation, diagnosis, and treatment. They can provide appropriate advice and guidance on integrating homeopathic remedies into your overall healthcare plan.

It's also important to communicate openly with your healthcare team about all the treatments and remedies that you are using, including any homeopathic remedies. This helps ensure they have a complete understanding of your healthcare choices and can provide the best possible care.

HOW DOES IT WORK?

By supporting the body's 'vital force', homeopathy works on an energetic level to activate the body's healing mechanisms, fostering a lasting state of wellness. While the scientific basis for homeopathy is still a subject of debate, some theories propose that homeopathic remedies may act through modulation of the body's neuroendocrine and immune systems or through the influence of subtle energy fields. Central to the philosophy of homeopathy is the concept of potentization, a process in which substances are diluted and then shaken vigorously (succussion) to release their energetic properties and minimize any potential toxicity. This dilution and succussion are believed to enhance the medicinal qualities of the substances, making them more effective and safer for use.

Mind body and soul

One of the unique aspects of homeopathy is its personal approach to treatment. With its emphasis on holistic a healing, considering the person rather than targeting specific symptoms, homeopathy has no single 'magic pill' that can be universally prescribed for a particular illness. No two patients are treated in the same way, as each person's symptom picture and constitution guide the selection of remedies. This highly individualized approach acknowledges the fact that different people may respond differently to the same illness, which is why treatment is tailored accordingly.

Homeopathy also recognises the huge effect that emotional and mental factors and have on physical ailments, and vice versa. Therefore, an in-depth analysis of the patient's overall state is considered crucial in homeopathic practice.

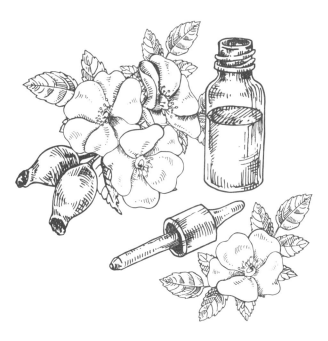

Another characteristic that distinguishes it from conventional medicine is its emphasis on self-healing. Rather than merely suppressing symptoms, the remedies aim to stimulate the body's innate healing abilities, empowering it to regain balance and fight off disease. This approach aligns with the concept of vitalism, which recognises the body's inherent life force and its capacity for self-regulation.

Homeopathy – the benefits

People use homeopathy for a variety of reasons, often seeking a natural and holistic approach to healthcare. Here are just some of them:

1. Gentle and non-toxic

Homeopathic remedies are made from highly diluted substances, making them gentle and safe for most individuals, including infants, children, and pregnant women. They are non-toxic and do not typically cause side effects or drug interactions.

2. Individualized treatment

Homeopathy emphasizes the individuality of each person, taking into account their unique symptoms, physical and emotional characteristics, and overall constitution.

Remedies are chosen based on the principle of 'like cures like,' where a substance that can produce symptoms in a healthy person is used to treat similar symptoms in a sick person.

3. Holistic approach

Homeopathy aims to treat the person as a whole, considering physical, mental, and emotional aspects. It recognizes the interconnectedness of symptoms and seeks to address the underlying imbalances rather than merely suppressing symptoms.

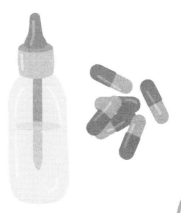

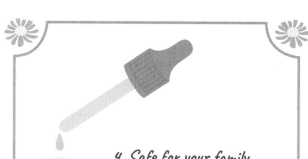

4. Safe for your family

Homeopathy is often considered a safe option for children since the remedies are highly diluted and generally well-tolerated.

5. Integrative care

Many people choose homeopathy as a complementary or alternative approach to conventional medicine. They may use homeopathy alongside conventional treatments to support overall health, alleviate symptoms, or reduce side effects of medications.

6. Chronic conditions

Homeopathy is often sought for chronic conditions, where conventional medicine may have limitations in providing long-term relief. It aims to stimulate the body's natural healing abilities, addressing the root cause of the imbalance and promoting overall well-being.

7. Patient-centred care

Homeopathic consultations typically involve a detailed assessment of the person's symptoms, medical history, and lifestyle factors. The focus is on understanding the individual and tailoring treatment to their specific needs, fostering a therapeutic and supportive patient-practitioner relationship.

CASE STUDY

Sarah's story

Homeopathy was 'absolutely life-changing' for Sarah's teenage son when he developed serious behavioural problems

"Luke is my middle child, and I knew from birth that there was something different about him. As a baby, he screamed non-stop and didn't meet any of the usual milestones. By the time he was two years old, I was really struggling to cope and made an appointment with a homeopath to help me manage my stress levels.

I took Luke with me to my first appointment with the homeopath and during the consultation, she said that she might also be able to help him. I was a bit sceptical, but she prescribed a remedy and within two days, Luke was like a different child. It was truly astounding.

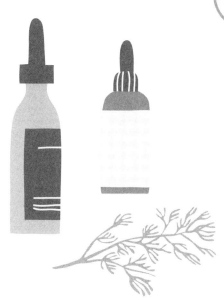

By this time, Luke had been diagnosed with autism but, with the help of the remedies, his behaviour was manageable and family life continued happily.

Violent tantrums

Then when Luke turned 14, things took a turn for the worse. During lockdown he'd become addicted to gaming. He was also showing hoarding behaviours and exhibiting signs of body dysmorphia. Whenever I tried to persuade him to come away from his PlayStation, he became violent, destroying furniture and punching walls.

Over the next six months, Luke's behaviour became increasingly worrying. He had violent tantrums, which sometimes went on for hours at a time. His brothers were scared of him and it was having a hugely negative impact on the whole family. Because Luke's behaviour was so extreme, it didn't occur to me that something as gentle as homeopathy could possibly help. But eventually I was so desperate that I called the homeopath. Because of lockdown, we had to do the consultation online but she prescribed Tuberculinum 200c and, within less than a week, Luke was once again a different person.

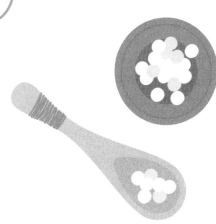

It saved our family

The tantrums stopped and the body dysmorphia and hoarding vanished. Luke wasn't even phased when his PlayStation broke! More than that, he became communicative and helpful. When he offered to make someone a sandwich—which would have been inconceivable before—I knew we'd really turned a corner!

I'm blown away by how powerful homeopathy can be. It's been absolutely life-changing."

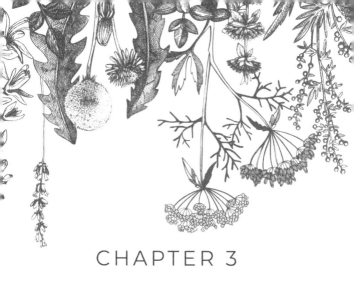

CHAPTER 3

Your Health

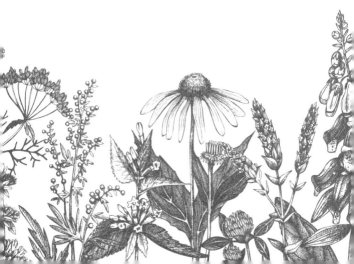

HOW ARE HOMEOPATHIC REMEDIES MADE?

Making these gentle healing remedies involves an intricate series of steps that are designed to extract the healing properties of the substance and transform it into a safe and effective remedy.

This begins with the selection of source materials, which can be plant, animal, or mineral substances. These substances are chosen based on their known properties and their ability to induce specific symptoms when administered to healthy individuals. For instance, plants like Arnica montana are used to treat bruising and muscle soreness, while minerals like Calcarea carbonica are employed for conditions like fatigue and sluggishness.

This source material is then finely ground and soaked in a mixture of alcohol and water to extract its medicinal properties. The resulting liquid is then filtered to remove any solid particles. This mixture is known as the mother tincture.

Potentization

The mother tincture is then diluted in a process called potentisation, which involves increasing the potency through a series of dilutions and succussions (shakings). These are designed to increase the healing properties of the remedy while reducing any potential side effects. The dilution process is typically done in a series of steps, with each step increasing the dilution level of the remedy. The level of dilution is indicated by a number, such as 6X or 30C. The X and C refer to the Roman numerals for 10 and 100, respectively. For example, a 6X remedy has been diluted one part mother tincture to nine parts diluent (usually water) six times, resulting in a total dilution of one part in one million.

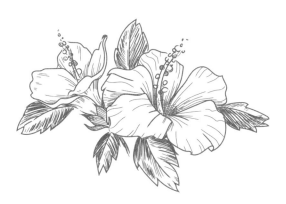

Vibrational healing

This final step in making a homeopathic remedy is to impregnate the dilutent with the energy or vibration of the original substance. This is done through a process called imprinting, in which the diluted remedy is exposed to the energy of the substance through succussion, the process of shaking or striking the remedy against a hard surface.

These succussions are an important part of the potentization process. Each dilution is shaken vigorously to energize the remedy and release its healing properties. The number of succussions can vary depending on the potency level of the remedy, with higher potency remedies requiring more succussions.

Energetic imprint

Remember that the dilution levels used in homeopathy are often extremely high. In fact, by the time a remedy reaches higher potencies such as 30C or beyond, it is highly unlikely that any molecules of the original substance remain in the solution. As per homeopathic philosophy, the succussion is believed to imprint the energetic properties of the substance onto the diluted solution. The homeopathic remedies are then dispensed as tiny sugar pellets or tablets, which have been saturated with the diluted solution. In some cases, liquid dilutions or ointments may also be used. These resulting remedies contain the healing energy of the original substance but are completely safe and free from any harmful side effects.

WHAT HAPPENS DURING A CONSULTATION?

During a homeopathic consultation, which can take up to 90 minutes, the homeopath will aim to understand your unique symptoms, overall health, and individual characteristics in order to prescribe the most suitable homeopathic remedy. Here's what typically happens during a homeopathic consultation:

Case Taking: The homeopath will begin by asking you detailed questions about your current symptoms, past medical history, lifestyle, emotional well-being, and any other relevant factors. They will listen attentively to your concerns and encourage you to provide as much information as possible. The questions may seem extensive and cover various aspects of your health and life.

Individualized Assessment: The homeopath will analyse the information you provide to gain insight into your specific patterns, modalities (factors that worsen or alleviate symptoms), and unique expression of the ailment. They will seek to understand the underlying causes and potential triggers for your symptoms.

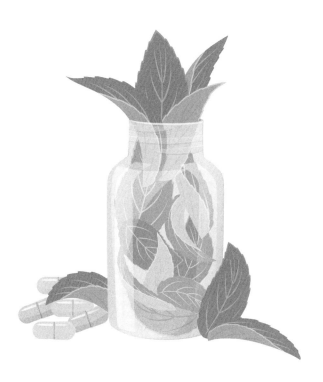

Holistic Evaluation: Homeopaths take a holistic approach, considering not only your physical symptoms but also your mental, emotional, and spiritual well-being. They will explore your personality traits, emotional responses, and how you experience and express your symptoms.

Remedy Selection: Based on the information gathered, the homeopath will match your symptoms and individual characteristics to the appropriate homeopathic remedy. Homeopathic remedies are derived from natural substances and are selected based on the principle of 'like cures like' — a substance that can produce symptoms in a healthy person can stimulate the body's healing response to similar symptoms in a sick person.

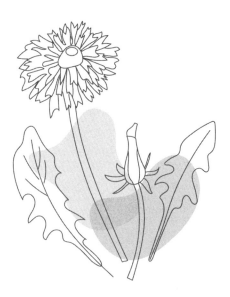

Treatment Plan: The homeopath will explain the selected remedy, its dosage, and how frequently it should be taken. They may also provide guidance on lifestyle modifications, dietary recommendations, and other supportive measures to enhance the healing process. The treatment plan will be tailored to your specific needs and may be adjusted over time based on your response and progress.

Follow-up Consultations: Homeopathy often involves multiple follow-up consultations to assess your progress, make any necessary adjustments to the remedy or dosage, and monitor your overall health. The frequency of follow-up visits may vary depending on the nature of your condition and individual circumstances.

It's important to note that homeopathy treats each person as an individual, so the same ailment may be addressed differently in different individuals. The duration of treatment can vary depending on the complexity and chronicity of the condition.

TEN QUESTIONS TO ASK

Lucy Godfrey of the charity Homeopathy UK outlines the questions you should ask if you are going to see a homeopath.

1. What qualifications do you have?

If a homeopath is registered with an organisation, then you can be reassured that they have been trained to a high standard, are fully qualified and are insured to treat patients. Each register has its own qualifications and homeopaths use the letters after their name to denote achievement.

2. How much do you charge?

Most homeopaths have fixed charges in the same way an acupuncturist or chiropractor does. The initial consultation normally costs more because it is longer.

3. What experience do you have treating my condition?

If the homeopath has treated many patients with your condition and has had success, they should be able to cite examples. However, homeopathy looks at you as a whole person and addresses your own body's ability to heal.

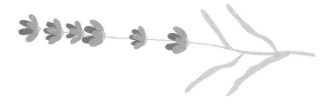

4. Do you accept private health insurance?

Some homeopaths are approved providers of
homeopathy through private insurance schemes.
You will need to ask the homeopath if they are
registered with your insurer.

5. How do you work and what should I expect from this consultation?

Each homeopath will have different operational
hours, set appointments, and style of service. At
the outset you should feel comfortable in how the
homeopath interacts with you and manages and
prioritises you as a patient. You should understand
clearly what the homeopath will be doing during
the consultation, how they will be charging you,
what the homeopath will be doing after your
appointment, when your next appointment is
scheduled for, and whether they will call you, etc.
For both parties it is best to be very clear and
comfortable with arrangements.

6. Will you write to my GP?

You will need to give your consent for your
homeopath to write to your GP and keep them
updated on your treatment. It is a good idea to
keep your GP in the picture and, if your treatment
is successful, they may be persuaded to refer
patients for homeopathy or even find out more
about it for themselves.

7. Should I stop taking my other medications and will homeopathy interfere with any of my current medications?

You should never stop any conventional
medication that has been prescribed by a doctor
without consulting them first. Homeopathy
can be taken alongside and in complement to
any conventional medication and there are no
known interactions. Homeopathy is free of side
effects and can even help with the side effects of
conventional medication.

8. What have you prescribed?

The homeopath should tell you what homeopathic
remedy they have prescribed.

9. What will happen after I take the homeopathic medicine?

The homeopath should clearly state in general terms the improvement they would expect to see over a few weeks. It is best to be clear about expectations and improvements, so that during the follow-up consultation, the homeopath can know what best to prescribe to maintain or improve your health.

10. How do I contact you in emergency?

Sometimes with a homeopathic prescription, symptoms can flare up but will settle again, however if you are having difficulties you need to know how or who to contact outside office hours. Ask the homeopath about this at your first consultation.

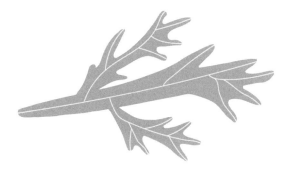

CHAPTER 4

Daily
Healing

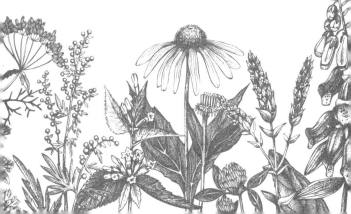

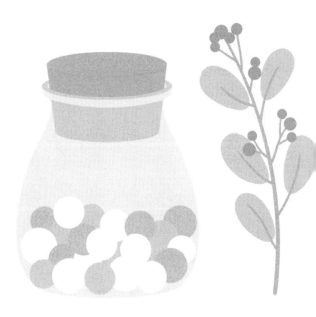

You can use homeopathic remedies in all aspects of your life, from raising a family, going on holiday, looking after your pets and dealing with exam stress and illness. The following chapter outlines some everyday situations and how homeopathy can offer gentle support.

HOMEOPATHY AND YOUR FAMILY

One of the advantages of homeopathy for children is that it is safe and gentle, with minimal risk of side effects, as it uses such diluted substances. In fact, homeopathy is commonly used to treat a wide range of health conditions in children, from common ailments like colds and ear infections to chronic conditions such as asthma and eczema. And research backs this up. For example, a randomized controlled trial published in the *British Medical Journal* showed that homeopathic treatment was effective in reducing the duration of diarrhoea in children. What's more, remedies are easy to administer as they usually come in the form of small pellets or liquid drops that are easy for children to take.

When using homeopathy for children, it's important to consult with a qualified homeopath or a healthcare professional trained in homeopathy. It's also important to follow the recommended dosages and guidelines provided by the homeopath as the dosages and frequencies of homeopathic remedies may vary depending on each individual case.

Chamomilla: Often used for teething issues, irritability, and restlessness in children. It can help soothe discomfort, calm fussiness, and promote better sleep. Chamomilla is typically administered in pellet form or as a diluted liquid, following the recommended dosage based on the child's age and symptoms.

Pulsatilla: Commonly used for children who are clingy, weepy, and seek comfort. It can be helpful for conditions like earaches, colds, and digestive disturbances. The remedy is usually given in pellet form or diluted liquid, following the dosage instructions specific to the child's age and symptoms.

Arnica: A well-known remedy for bumps, bruises, and muscle soreness. It can be used after falls or minor injuries to reduce swelling, pain, and promote healing. Arnica is available in pellet form or as a topical cream or gel for external application.

Aconite: For sudden onset fevers, fright, and restlessness. It can be beneficial during the early stages of colds, flu, or other acute illnesses. Aconite is typically administered in pellet form or diluted liquid, following the appropriate dosage instructions based on the child's age and symptoms.

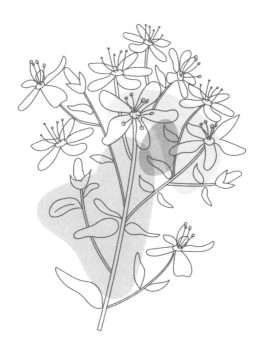

Calcarea carbonica: Commonly used for children who are slow to develop, have a tendency towards obesity, and have trouble in adapting to change. It can help with issues like slow growth, digestive complaints, and recurrent infections. The dosage and potency will vary depending on the child's age and symptoms.

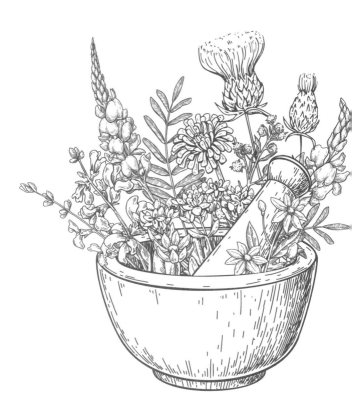

Your Homeopathic Kit

Create a handy holistic kit filled with gentle homeopathic remedies for minor illnesses and injuries. Use it alongside your regular first aid kit, which should include essentials like bandages, gauze, tape, scissors, tweezers, antiseptic and a thermometer. Remember, it's important to store your remedies in a cool, dry place away from sunlight and strong odours.

Here are some common remedies and items you might consider including in your kit:

Arnica montana

This remedy is useful for treating bruises, muscle soreness, and strains. It can be taken orally or applied topically in the form of creams, gels, or ointments.

Calendula officinalis

Great for promoting wound healing and can be used topically in the form of creams, gels, or ointments.

Hypericum perforatum

Often used for nerve pain and injuries to sensitive areas, such as fingers and toes. It can be taken orally or applied topically in the form of creams, gels, or ointments.

Belladonna

Often used for sudden onset fever, redness, and inflammation. It can be taken orally in pellet or liquid form.

Aconitum napellus

Useful for treating sudden onset cold and flu symptoms, especially if there is a fever. It can be taken orally in pellet or liquid form.

Apis mellifica

Helpful for treating insect bites and stings, as well as allergic reactions. It can be taken orally in pellet or liquid form.

Ledum palustre

Great for treating puncture wounds and animal bites. It can be taken orally in pellet or liquid form.

Nux vomica

Good for digestive upsets, such as nausea, vomiting, and diarrhoea. It can be taken orally in pellet or liquid form.

Rescue Remedy

This is a blend of several remedies and is useful for acute stress, shock, and emotional trauma. It can be taken orally in pellet or liquid form.

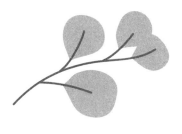

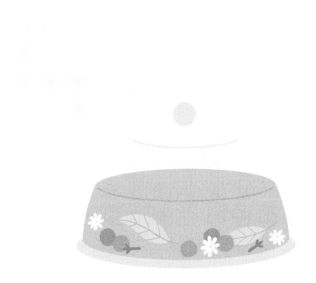

FEELING STRESSED?

Homeopathy can be helpful in managing different types of stressful and emotionally charged situations by addressing both the associated physical and emotional symptoms. Here are some common stressful situations and corresponding homeopathic remedies that may provide relief:

Grief and Loss

Ignatia amara can be effective for acute grief, sadness, and emotional upheaval, especially after the loss of a loved one or a significant life change while Natrum muriaticum can be useful for chronic grief, feelings of isolation, and a tendency to suppress emotions.

Exam Anxiety

Argentum nitricum can help with anticipatory anxiety, nervousness, and performance anxiety before exams while Gelsemium sempervirens is helpful for exam-related anxiety with trembling, weakness, and mental fatigue.

Public Speaking

Lycopodium clavatum can help with stage fright, lack of confidence, and fear of public speaking while Silicea can help with nervousness, and fear of failure during public speaking.

Performance Anxiety

Gelsemium sempervirens is helpful for trembling, weakness, and anticipatory anxiety before performances while Lycopodium clavatum is useful for lack of self-confidence, fear of failure, and stage fright.

Work-related Stress

Nux vomica is effective for stress from long working hours, excessive ambition, and irritability while Sepia can help for work-related stress with fatigue, indifference, and feeling overwhelmed.

Relationship Stress

Ignatia amara is useful for grief, emotional turmoil, and sensitivity to relationship stress while Natrum muriaticum is helpful for suppressed emotions, sadness, and isolation in response to relationship stress.

Financial Stress

Calcarea carbonica can help people who feel overwhelmed and anxious about financial matters, particularly when associated with overwork and exhaustion while Staphysagria is useful for suppressed anger and frustration due to financial stress, especially when it involves feeling undermined or taken advantage of.

Social Anxiety

Lycopodium clavatum can help people with low self-confidence, fear of judgment, and avoidance of social situations while Phosphorus can help with social anxiety characterised by fear of public scrutiny, excessive sensitivity, and a strong desire for companionship.

Fear of Heights

Baryta carbonica can help people who experience fear and insecurity when confronted with heights, especially in unfamiliar or exposed situations while Gelsemium sempervirens is helpful for anticipatory anxiety and trembling when faced with heights or the thought of heights.

Claustrophobia

Arsenicum album can help with anxiety, restlessness, and fear experienced in enclosed or tight space while Pulsatilla can help people who feel anxious and panicky in confined spaces but find relief when given reassurance and open spaces.

Agoraphobia

Aconitum napellus is useful for sudden panic attacks, restlessness, and fear of being in crowded or open spaces while Argentum nitricum can help people with anxiety, nervousness, and fear of public places, especially when accompanied by anticipation of negative outcomes.

CASE STUDY

CASE STUDY

Anne's story

Anne tackled her fear of heights with homeopathy

"I can remember exactly when I first experienced acrophobia. I had taken my daughter to the ballet at Sadler's Wells and booked my favourite seats—first row dress circle. What I hadn't bargained for was the steepness of the tiering. I sat down and couldn't move for fear that I would topple over the balcony. Although I knew intellectually that this was totally improbable, I couldn't stop the feelings.

That day was a turning point. I went from someone who loved high and scary fairground rides to being riveted to the spot through fear. At these times, my insides felt as though they were going to fall out—not a very pleasant feeling. On holidays, high balconies were a misery and sight-seeing was often curtailed. Going down a steep escalator on the underground was a torment. And I became increasingly worried about falling down stairs.

I was clinging to the walls

Over the next few years, my acrophobia increased in severity. The Eiffel Tower and Notre Dame left me clinging to walls. Sitting in the upper circle at the theatre, I knew that if someone had placed a million pounds in front of me, I would not have been able to pick it up for fear of toppling over. During the interval, I was only able to leave my seat when a kind man, seeing my terror,

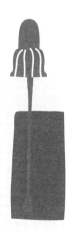

held me as I made my way along the row. I didn't return for the second act.

Acrophobia isn't a debilitating disease, but it was having a major effect on my social life. I decided the time had come to contact an expert and reached out to a homeopath. He suggested taking one 30c Lac Felinum half an hour before going into a theatre (or anywhere where I had problems) and then one as needed throughout the performance.

During my next theatre trip, I had to take the remedy several times during the performance, but the fact that I'd managed to stay in my seat meant it was working. A few weeks later I was absolutely fine, even though I was sitting in the gods!"

Anne Coates is the author of the Hannah Weybridge crimes thrillers, Dancers in the Wind, Death's Silent Judgement, Songs of Innocents, Perdition's Child and Stage Call.

ON HOLIDAY

Going on holiday and have a terrible fear of flying? Or maybe you just want to avoid getting an upset stomach in a new environment? Homeopathic remedies can be brilliant travel companions when you're on the move. Here are a few firm favourites:

Jet Lag

Remedies like Arnica montana, Cocculus indicus, and Nux vomica can help alleviate the symptoms of jet lag, such as fatigue, disrupted sleep patterns, and disorientation.

Travel Sickness

Remedies like Cocculus indicus can help with nausea, dizziness, and motion sickness during travel while Tabacum can soothe intense nausea, cold sweats, and pale skin associated with travel sickness.

Fear of Flying:

Try Aconitum napellus, which is useful for anxiety, restlessness, and fear before or during flights or Gelsemium sempervirens for anticipatory anxiety, trembling, and weakness related to flying.

Sunburn

Calendula officinalis and Cantharis are commonly used remedies for sunburn. They can be applied topically in a diluted form or taken internally to promote healing.

Insect bites and stings

Apis mellifica, Ledum palustre, and Urtica urens are some commonly used remedies that can help relieve itching, swelling, and pain associated with insect bites and stings.

Digestive issues

Changes in diet, eating unfamiliar foods, or consuming contaminated food and water while travelling can lead to digestive issues such as diarrhoea, indigestion, or food poisoning. Homeopathic remedies like Arsenicum album, Nux vomica, and Veratrum album can be useful in addressing these symptoms.

Homesickness

Travelling can sometimes bring about emotional stress, anxiety, or homesickness. Remedies such as Ignatia amara, Pulsatilla, and Lycopodium can help support emotional well-being and balance during these times.

Insomnia or sleep disturbances

Adjusting to a new environment or time zone can disrupt sleep patterns. Homeopathic remedies like Coffea cruda, Passiflora incarnata, and Kali phosphoricum can aid in promoting better sleep and addressing insomnia.

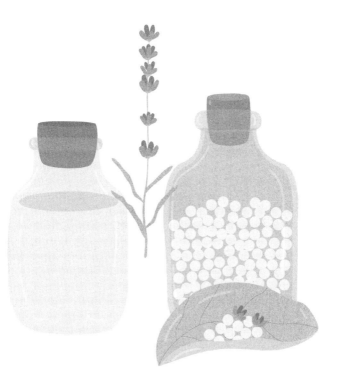

HOMEOPATHY AND YOUR PETS

Homeopathy can be a safe and effective treatment option for animals as well as humans. Research shows that the basic principles of homeopathy apply to animals just as they do to humans. For example, a randomized controlled trial published in the *Journal of Veterinary Internal Medicine* found that homeopathic treatment was effective in reducing the severity of diarrhoea in dogs. Meanwhile, in a laboratory setting, research published in the journal *Inflammation Research* showed that it reduced inflammation in rats, indicating a potential anti-inflammatory effect. When administering homeopathic remedies to pets, it's important to use the correct dosage and potency. Consult with a veterinarian trained in homeopathy for guidance on how to properly administer remedies to your pet. It's also important to monitor your pet's symptoms and response to the remedy, and to seek veterinary care if symptoms persist or worsen.

Here are some common homeopathic remedies and their uses in pets:

Arnica

Commonly used to relieve pain and inflammation associated with injuries, such as sprains, bruises, and muscle soreness. It can be used topically or orally.

Belladonna

Can be used to relieve fever, inflammation, and pain in pets, particularly when these symptoms are sudden and intense.

Chamomilla

Can be helpful for pets that are agitated or irritable, particularly if they are experiencing pain or discomfort. It can also be used to relieve digestive upset.

Nux vomica

Often used to relieve gastrointestinal symptoms, such as vomiting, diarrhoea, and constipation. It can also be helpful for pets that are irritable or have difficulty relaxing.

Pulsatilla

Can be used to relieve respiratory symptoms, such as coughing and wheezing, as well as digestive upset and ear infections.

CASE STUDY

Melanie's story

Melanie used homeopathy to treat her dog Eddy when he became ill

"My husband Joe and I had adopted Eddy—a German Shepherd/Lab cross—as a stray. Eddy suffered from genetic hip issues and his joints became so malformed that he shouldn't have been able to walk. Joe's father was a homeopath, so he prescribed a remedy for Eddy, who was able to stay mobile and even managed a walk on the day he passed away. It really was a miracle that he didn't have to have an op, or even worse, lose the use of his legs.

We also successfully used homeopathy to treat a bout of distemper when Eddy was a puppy. Despite being a very young dog, the vet said that there was nothing he could do, and Eddy would need to be put down.

We were devastated but, once again Joe's father stepped in and, once again, Eddy responded amazingly well to the remedy. Thanks to the various homeopathic treatments, Eddy went on to live until the ripe old age of 17."

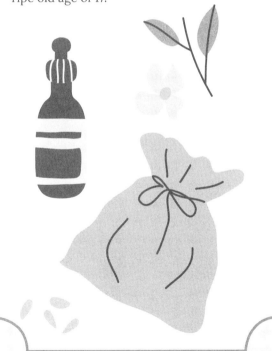

DIY HOMEOPATHIC RECIPES

Making your own homeopathic remedies is an excellent way to treat minor stresses and ailments at home. Here are a few to try:

Arnica oil: Arnica is used for treating bruises, sprains, and muscle soreness. You can make this soothing oil by mixing dried arnica flowers with a carrier oil like olive oil or almond oil. Allow the mixture to infuse for several weeks, strain, and use as needed.

Calendula cream: Calendula is known for its healing properties and is commonly used for skin irritations, cuts, and burns. You can make gentle cream by combining calendula-infused oil with beeswax, shea butter, and essential oils like lavender or tea tree oil.

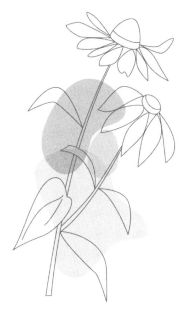

Echinacea tincture: Echinacea is believed to boost the immune system and help prevent and treat colds and flu. Prepare this health-boosting tincture by steeping dried echinacea root in alcohol for several weeks and then straining the liquid.

Chamomile tea: Chamomile is used for promoting relaxation, reducing anxiety, and improving sleep. You can make this calming drink by steeping chamomile flowers in hot water for several minutes.

Ginger tea: Ginger is known for its anti-inflammatory and digestive properties. Make this warming tea by steeping fresh ginger root in hot water for several minutes, and then adding honey and lemon to taste.

Hypericum oil: Hypericum is used for nerve pain and injuries. Infuse dried Hypericum perforatum (St John's wort) flowers in a carrier oil like olive oil or coconut oil for several weeks, strain, and use topically as needed.

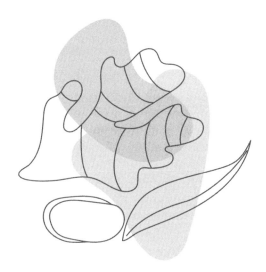

Nux vomica remedy: Nux vomica is used for digestive issues like indigestion and heartburn. Dilute Nux vomica 6C or 30C potency in water according to the instructions on the remedy vial, and take it orally as directed.

Rhus tox lotion: Rhus toxicodendron (poison ivy) is used for joint and muscle pain. Create a lotion by diluting Rhus tox mother tincture or a low potency (e.g. 6X) in water or aloe vera gel, and apply topically to the affected area.

Aconite throat spray: Aconitum napellus is used for sore throats and the early stages of colds or flu. Dilute Aconite mother tincture or a low potency (e.g. 6C) in water, and use it as a throat spray.

Plantain salve: Plantain is used for skin irritations, insect bites, and minor wounds. Infuse dried plantain leaves in a carrier oil, strain, and combine with beeswax to create a healing salve.

Belladonna compress: Belladonna is used for fever and inflammatory conditions. Dilute Belladonna mother tincture or a low potency (e.g. 6C) in water, soak a cloth in the solution, and apply it as a compress to reduce inflammation.

Sepia facial mask: Sepia is used for hormonal imbalances and skin issues. Mix Sepia 6C or 30C potency with water and apply it as a facial mask to address skin concerns.

Silicea powder for nails: Silicea is used for brittle nails. Dissolve Silicea 6X or 12X potency tablets in water and soak your nails in the solution to help strengthen them.

Cantharis ointment: Cantharis is used for burns and bladder irritation. Combine Cantharis mother tincture or a low potency (e.g., 6C) with a carrier ointment like petroleum jelly, and apply it topically to burns or skin irritations.

Kali phosphoricum toner: Kali phosphoricum is used for mental and physical exhaustion. Dissolve Kali phos 6X or 30X potency tablets in water and use the solution as a facial toner for revitalisation.

Bryonia syrup for cough: Bryonia alba is used for dry, irritating coughs. Make a syrup by dissolving Bryonia 6C or 30C potency pellets in water and adding raw honey. Take small spoonfuls as needed for cough relief.

Ignatia eye drops for eye strain: Ignatia amara is used for eye strain and emotional stress. Dissolve Ignatia 6X or 30X potency pellets in distilled water and use the solution as eye drops to alleviate strain and discomfort.

Pulsatilla steam for congestion: Pulsatilla is used for nasal congestion. Boil water in a pot, add a few drops of Pulsatilla mother tincture or a low potency (e.g. 6C) to the water, and inhale the steam to help relieve congestion.

Chamomilla teething gel: Chamomilla is used for teething pain in infants and children. Combine Chamomilla mother tincture or a low potency (e.g. 6C) with a carrier gel like aloe vera gel and apply it to the gums for soothing relief.

Ruta graveolens balm for sprains: Ruta graveolens is used for sprains and strains. Infuse dried Ruta graveolens leaves in a carrier oil like olive oil or coconut oil, strain, and mix with beeswax to create a healing balm for topical application.

Top 50 homeopathic remedies

1. **Aconitum napellus:** Sudden onset of high fever, anxiety, restlessness.
2. **Arnica montana:** Trauma, bruises, muscle soreness.
3. **Belladonna:** High fever, throbbing headache, inflammation.
4. **Bryonia alba:** Dry cough, joint pains aggravated by motion.
5. **Calendula officinalis:** Wounds, cuts, burns, skin infections.
6. **Chamomilla:** Teething problems, irritability, colic in infants.
7. **Coffea cruda:** Sleeplessness due to mental overactivity.
8. **Colocynthis:** Abdominal cramps, colic, sciatica.
9. **Drosera rotundifolia:** Spasmodic cough, hoarseness.
10. **Gelsemium sempervirens:** Flu-like symptoms, weakness, trembling.

11. **Ginkgo biloba:** cognitive function, memory and circulation.

12. **Hepar sulphuris calcareum:** Abscesses, infections, croupy cough.

13. **Hypericum perforatum:** Nerve injuries, shooting pains.

14. **Ignatia amara:** Grief, emotional shock, hysteria.

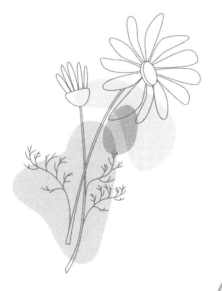

15. **Ipecacuanha:** Nausea, vomiting, persistent cough.

16. **Kali bichromicum:** Sinusitis, thick nasal discharge.

17. **Lachesis muta:** Hot flashes, left-sided symptoms, throat infections.

18. **Ledum palustre:** Insect bites, puncture wounds, gout.

19. **Lycopodium clavatum:** Digestive issues, bloating, liver ailments.

20. **Mercurius solubilis:** Sore throat, excessive salivation, sweating.

21. **Natrum muriaticum:** Emotional stress, grief, headaches.

22. **Nux vomica:** Indigestion, hangover, irritability.

23. **Phosphorus:** Respiratory issues, haemorrhages, anxiety.

24. **Phytolacca decandra:** Sore throat, breast inflammation.

25. **Pulsatilla nigricans:** Hormonal imbalances, weepiness, digestive problems.

26. **Rhus toxicodendron:** Joint stiffness, sprains, restless legs.
27. **Ruta graveolens:** Tendonitis, eye strain, bruises.
28. **Sepia officinalis:** Hormonal imbalances, fatigue, indifference.
29. **Silicea:** Abscesses, brittle nails, lack of stamina.
30. **Spongia tosta:** Croup, dry cough, thyroid issues.
31. **Staphysagria:** Surgical incisions, suppressed anger, urinary issues.
32. **Sulphur:** Skin conditions, hot flashes, itching.
33. **Symphytum officinale:** Bone injuries, fractures, eye injuries.
34. **Thuja occidentalis:** Skin growths, warts, urinary issues.
35. **Aesculus hippocastanum:** Haemorrhoids, venous congestion.
36. **Agaricus muscarius:** Nerve pain, twitching, trembling.

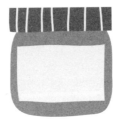

37. **Allium cepa:** Allergic rhinitis, watery eyes, runny nose.
38. **Antimonium tartaricum:** Bronchitis, rattling cough, chest congestion.
39. **Apis mellifica:** Insect bites, allergic reactions, swollen joints.
40. **Argentum nitricum:** Anxiety, anticipatory fears, digestive issues.
41. **Baptisia tinctoria:** Flu, septic conditions, foul breath.
42. **Calcarea carbonica:** Slow development, weak bones, cold intolerance.
43. **Carbo vegetabilis:** Gas, bloating, indigestion.

44. **Causticum:** Urinary incontinence, hoarseness, muscle weakness.
45. **Cimicifuga racemosa:** Menstrual cramps, emotional instability.
46. **Digitalis purpurea:** Heart conditions, irregular pulse.
47. **Dulcamara:** Allergies, joint pain worsened by damp weather.
48. **Eupatorium perfoliatum:** Influenza, bone pains, dengue fever.
49. **Ferrum phosphoricum:** Fever, inflammation, anaemia.
50. **Veratrum album:** Diarrhoea, vomiting, collapse.

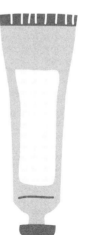

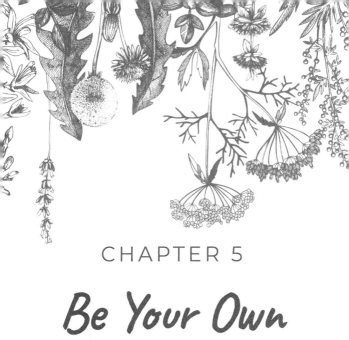

CHAPTER 5

Be Your Own Homeopath

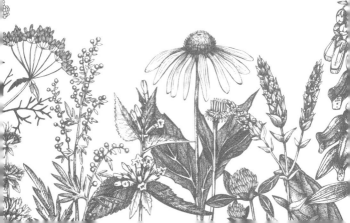

You can treat yourself with homeopathy in some situations as the remedies are generally safe and you can buy them over the counter at some health food stores, pharmacies, and online. However, do bear in mind that self-treatment may not be appropriate for chronic or complex conditions that require a comprehensive evaluation and individualized treatment plan. Remember that while treating

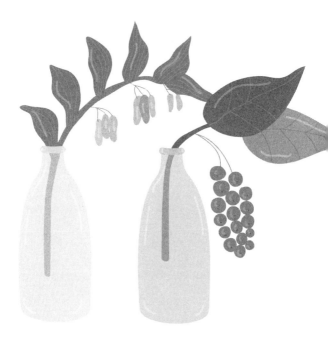

yourself can be effective with certain acute health complaints, it does have its limitations and you should always seek guidance from a qualified homeopath for more complex or chronic conditions who can provide personalized guidance and monitor your progress over time.

Here are some general guidelines for using DIY homeopathic remedies:

Acute conditions: Acute conditions are self-limiting diseases which start quickly and are usually of short duration. Homeopathy is well-suited for self-treatment of minor acute conditions, such as common colds, bruises, minor injuries, indigestion, or mild allergies as it can help to alleviate symptoms and promote the body's natural healing process.

Familiarity with remedies: It's helpful to have some knowledge of common homeopathic remedies and their indications. Use this book as your first point of reference.

Match symptoms: To select the most appropriate remedy, it's important to match your symptoms as closely as possible to the indications of the remedy. Homeopathic remedies are chosen based on the principle of 'like cures like', where a substance that can cause symptoms in a healthy person is used to treat similar symptoms in an individual with an illness.

Choose the correct remedy: Homeopathic remedies are selected based on individual symptoms and characteristics. Research the specific symptoms you are experiencing or seek guidance from a homeopath to determine the most appropriate remedy. Ideally you want to match three characteristic symptoms of the remedy (keynotes). Particular attention should be given to any mental or emotional symptoms.

Select the potency: Homeopathic remedies are available in different potencies (e.g. 6C, 30C, 200C). The potency selection depends on the severity of symptoms and individual response. It is generally recommended to start with lower potencies for self-use (6C and 30C). Potentising, as mentioned earlier, combines several serial dilutions of an original substance with vigorous shaking, known as succussion.

Follow dosage instructions: Homeopathic remedies are typically taken in pellet, tablet, or liquid form. They are highly diluted and often administered orally. Follow the dosage instructions provided with the remedy or consult a homeopath for guidance. Dosage frequency may vary, but it is common to take remedies multiple times a day initially and then reduce frequency as symptoms improve. For acute conditions homeopathic medicines are prescribed one at a time.

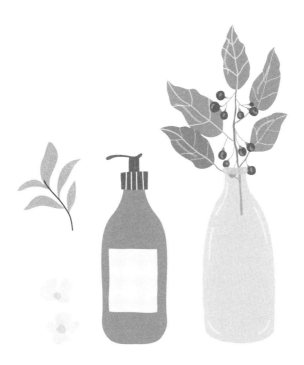

Administer properly: Avoid touching the remedies with your hands to prevent contamination. Use a clean spoon, place the remedy under your tongue, and let it dissolve. Avoid eating or drinking anything for about 15 minutes before and after taking the remedy, as certain substances can interfere with its absorption.

Monitor your response: Observe any changes in your symptoms, both improvements and aggravations. Keep a journal to track your progress. If symptoms worsen or persist, consult a homeopath for reassessment and possible adjustment of the remedy or potency. Usually the correct remedy will help very quickly.

Store Properly: Homeopathic remedies are sensitive to external factors such as heat, strong odours, and electromagnetic fields. Store them in a cool, dry place away from direct sunlight, strong odours, and electronic devices.

Common health complaints

The following remedies can be taken in a 30C potency, and it's generally suggested to take three to five pellets under the tongue, allowing them to dissolve.

Remember that self-prescribing homeopathic remedies may have limitations, especially for complex or chronic conditions. Professional guidance is recommended for an accurate diagnosis and appropriate remedy selection.

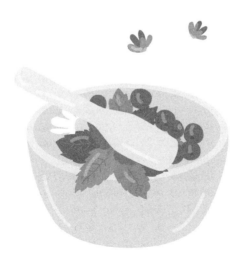

ALLERGIES

Allergies are the result of an overreactive immune response to substances that are typically harmless, such as pollen, dust mites, pet dander, or certain foods. When a person with allergies encounters these substances, their immune system identifies them as threats and releases chemicals like histamine, leading to symptoms such as sneezing, itching, watery eyes, and congestion. The exact cause of allergies is not fully understood, but genetic factors, environmental triggers, and immune system abnormalities are believed to play a role.

Homeopathy offers a holistic approach to treating allergies by stimulating the body's self-healing mechanisms and restoring balance. The remedies work by utilising highly diluted substances that, in larger doses, would cause similar symptoms to those experienced during an allergic reaction. This approach is believed to stimulate the body's vital force and encourage the immune system to rebalance itself.

Homeopathic helpers

Allium cepa: Indicated for allergic rhinitis with watery, burning nasal discharge and tearing, irritated eyes. Symptoms are often worse in warm rooms and improve in open air.

Euphrasia: Helpful for allergies with watery, acrid discharge from the eyes, along with burning and swelling. The eyes may be sensitive to light.

Natrum muriaticum: Suitable for nasal allergies with clear nasal discharge, sneezing, and a loss of taste or smell. Individuals needing Natrum muriaticum may have a craving for salt.

Sabadilla: Indicated for hay fever symptoms, including sneezing, itchy nose, red and watery eyes, and a tickling cough. Symptoms are often worse from the smell of flowers.

Arsenicum album: Useful for allergies with symptoms of nasal congestion, sneezing, and watery discharge, as well as burning and itching of the eyes and nose. Symptoms may worsen at night.

ARTHRITIS AND RHEUMATISM

Arthritis and rheumatism are both conditions that affect the joints and cause pain, inflammation, and stiffness. While they share similar symptoms, they have different underlying causes.

Arthritis is a general term used to describe inflammation of the joints. There are different types of arthritis, including osteoarthritis (caused by wear and tear of the joint cartilage), rheumatoid arthritis (an autoimmune disease), gout (caused by the build-up of uric acid crystals in the joints), and others. The causes of arthritis can vary depending on the specific type but may involve factors such as genetic predisposition, joint injuries, infections, immune system dysfunction, or metabolic abnormalities.

Rheumatism is a more general term that refers to a variety of painful conditions affecting the joints, muscles, tendons, and other soft tissues. It is often associated with generalized pain, stiffness, and inflammation. The causes of rheumatism are diverse and can include factors such as autoimmune diseases, chronic infections, hormonal imbalances, or environmental triggers.

Homeopathic helpers

Rhus toxicodendron: Indicated for arthritis and rheumatism with stiffness and pain that worsens upon initial movement but improves with continued motion. The affected joints may feel hot, swollen, and better with warmth and gentle stretching.

Bryonia: This remedy is used for arthritis with intense, stitching pain that worsens with movement. The affected joints may feel hot, swollen, and worse from even slight touch or motion.

Arnica: Helpful for joint pain and stiffness that result from injuries or overexertion. It is commonly used for arthritic conditions accompanied by soreness and bruised sensations in the joints.

Pulsatilla: Suitable for shifting pains in the joints that migrate from one joint to another. The pain is worse in the evening, with heat, and relieved by cold applications and gentle movement.

Calcarea carbonica: Indicated for arthritis with a sensation of coldness and stiffness in the joints. The pain is worse during damp weather and at the onset of movement but improves with continued motion.

ASTHMA

Asthma is a chronic respiratory condition characterized by inflammation and narrowing of the airways, resulting in symptoms such as wheezing, coughing, shortness of breath, and chest tightness. While asthma is a complex condition that requires medical management, homeopathy can help by providing complementary support in managing symptoms and improving overall well-being.

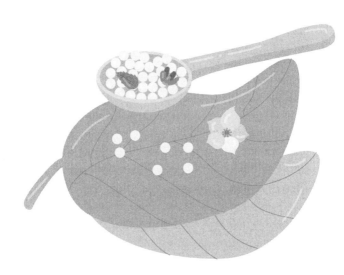

Homeopathic helpers

Arsenicum album: This remedy is indicated for asthma attacks that are accompanied by anxiety, restlessness and a sense of suffocation. Wheezing and coughing may worsen at night or with cold air exposure.

Natrum sulphuricum: Useful for asthma triggered by dampness or changes in weather. Wheezing, coughing, and difficulty breathing may be worse in humid environments.

Spongia tosta: Indicated for a dry, barking cough and wheezing that worsens with excitement or talking. Breathing may feel better when leaning forward.

Ipecacuanha: This remedy is recommended for asthma with persistent coughing, wheezing, and difficulty breathing. Coughing fits may be accompanied by vomiting or a feeling of nausea.

Antimonium tartaricum: Useful for asthma with rattling mucus in the chest, difficulty expectorating, and a sensation of suffocation. Breathing may be rapid and shallow.

BACK PAIN

This common health complaint can have various causes, including muscle strain, poor posture, herniated discs, arthritis or underlying medical conditions. Homeopathy can provide supportive care for back pain by addressing the underlying causes and promoting natural healing. Homeopathic remedies should complement appropriate medical care and be part of a comprehensive treatment plan. Additionally, lifestyle modifications, such as maintaining good posture, regular exercise and proper ergonomics, may also be important in managing back pain effectively.

Homeopathic helpers

Arnica: This remedy is often used for acute back pain resulting from injury or overexertion. It can help reduce pain, swelling, and bruising. Arnica is commonly available in gel or cream form for topical application.

Rhus toxicodendron: When back pain is worse on initial movement and improves with continued motion, Rhus toxicodendron may be considered. It is often used for back pain resulting from strains, sprains, or overexertion.

Bryonia: This remedy is suitable for sharp, stitching, or tearing pains that worsen with movement. The person may prefer lying still and applying pressure to the affected area. Bryonia is often used for back pain aggravated by even slight motion.

Kali carbonicum: When back pain is accompanied by weakness or a sensation of heaviness, Kali carbonicum may be helpful. It is often used for back pain worsened by sitting or lying down and improved by walking or bending backward.

Nux vomica: This remedy is commonly used for back pain caused by overexertion, prolonged sitting, or a sedentary lifestyle. The pain is often described as aching or cramping, and there may be associated digestive disturbances or irritability.

BLADDER PROBLEMS

Bladder problems can have various causes, including infections, inflammation, bladder muscle dysfunction, nerve damage, hormonal imbalances and structural abnormalities. Common bladder problems include urinary tract infections (UTIs), interstitial cystitis, overactive bladder, urinary incontinence and bladder stones. Homeopathy can be beneficial in addressing various bladder problems by considering your specific symptoms and overall health. It aims to stimulate the body's self-healing mechanism and restore balance.

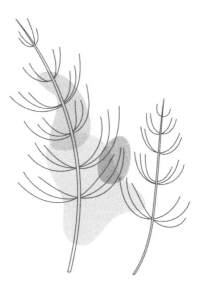

Homeopathic helpers

Cantharis: This remedy is often used for bladder infections and UTIs. It helps alleviate symptoms such as burning pain during urination and an intense urge to urinate.

Equisetum: Equisetum is commonly used for urinary problems such as a constant urge to urinate and discomfort in the bladder region. It may be helpful for conditions like interstitial cystitis.

Staphysagria: This remedy is often indicated for bladder problems that arise after suppression of the urge to urinate, such as from holding urine for extended periods. It may be useful for conditions like urinary incontinence.

Causticum: Causticum is frequently used for bladder problems associated with urinary incontinence, especially when laughing or coughing. It can also help with a weak urine flow.

Sepia: Sepia is often prescribed for bladder problems in women, particularly after childbirth, when there is a sensation of a weakened bladder or involuntary urine leakage.

BUMPS AND BRUISES

One of the most common health complaints, especially amongst children, homeopathy can help to promote faster healing and reducing painful symptoms. It's important to note that for severe injuries or head trauma, seeking immediate medical attention is essential. However, for mild to moderate bruises and bumps, homeopathy is a great healer. Additionally, rest, applying cold compresses or ice packs, and keeping the affected area elevated can speed up the healing process.

Homeopathic helpers

Arnica: Arnica is one of the most well-known remedies for bruises and trauma. It can help reduce swelling, pain, and discoloration associated with bruises. Arnica is often available in various forms, such as cream, gel, or pellets, and can be applied topically or taken orally.

Bellis perennis: This remedy is indicated for deep bruises or injuries to soft tissues, such as muscles or breasts. It can help reduce swelling, pain, and promote healing.

Ledum palustre: It is useful for puncture wounds or bruises caused by sharp objects, such as insect bites or stings. Ledum can help reduce swelling, discoloration, and alleviate pain.

Hamamelis: This remedy is helpful for bruises accompanied by venous congestion or varicose veins. It can help reduce swelling, bruising, and promote circulation in the affected area.

Symphytum: This is useful for bone bruises or injuries. Symphytum can aid in bone healing, reduce pain, and support the recovery process.

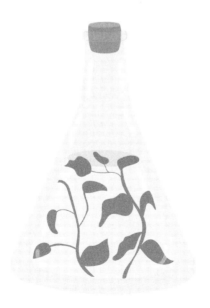

BURNS

When your skin is burned, it undergoes various physiological changes depending on the severity of the burn. Common symptoms include pain, redness, swelling, blistering and, in severe cases, skin damage or charring. For mild to moderate burns homeopathy can help support the healing process and alleviate symptoms but it's essential to seek medical attention for severe burns or those that involve a large area of the body. Additionally, follow general first aid measures for burns, such as cooling the burn with cool running water and covering it with a clean cloth.

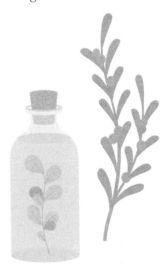

Homeopathic helpers

Cantharis: This remedy is often recommendedfor burns with intense burning pain and blistering. It can help alleviate pain, promote healing, and reduce the risk of infection.

Calendula: It is commonly used for its wound-healing properties. Calendula can be applied topically as a cream or diluted in water for washing the affected area. It helps soothe the skin, reduce inflammation, and promote the natural healing process.

Urtica urens: This remedy is helpful for burns with a stinging or prickling sensation, similar to a nettle sting. It can help relieve pain, reduce inflammation, and aid in the healing process.

Hypericum: This is indicated for burns involving nerve damage or intense pain. Hypericum can help alleviate pain, especially when the burn affects nerve-rich areas.

Arnica: This remedy may be considered for burns accompanied by bruising or trauma to the skin. Arnica can help reduce swelling, bruising, and promote tissue healing.

CHRONIC FATIGUE SYNDROME

Also known as Myalgic Encephalomyelitis (ME), Chronic Fatigue Syndrome (CFS) is a complex and debilitating disorder characterised by persistent fatigue that is not alleviated by rest and is accompanied by a range of other symptoms. The exact cause of CFS is unknown, but it is believed to be multifactorial, involving triggers such as viral or bacterial infections, immune system dysfunction, hormonal imbalances and psychological or emotional factors.

While homeopathy cannot cure this chronic condition, it can help by addressing underlying imbalances and support the body's self-healing capacity. Treatment requires a highly individualized approach so consulting with a qualified homeopath is recommended.

Homeopathic helpers

Gelsemium: Indicated for fatigue with weakness and heaviness of the limbs. There may be mental and physical exhaustion, drowsiness, and trembling. Symptoms worsen with emotional excitement or anticipation.

Kali phosphoricum: Helpful for mental and physical exhaustion with weakness, depression, and lack of motivation. Individuals may have trouble concentrating and have a sensation of heaviness or weakness in the limbs.

Phosphoric acid: Suitable for fatigue following emotional or physical exertion, grief, or prolonged stress. There may be mental and physical exhaustion, memory problems, and apathy.

Selenium: Indicated for weakness and fatigue with debility and exhaustion after illness or excessive physical exertion. There may be mental and physical weakness, tremors, and sensitivity to noise.

Picric acid: Useful for profound mental and physical exhaustion with extreme fatigue, especially after intellectual or physical exertion. Individuals may experience brain fog, difficulty concentrating, and headaches.

CASE STUDY

Janice's story

Janice used homeopathy to help with her chronic fatigue and mobility issues

"When I was a student, I was involved in a bad car crash. I was crossing the road when a drunk driver raced through a red traffic light. I went over the top of the car and although nothing was broken, I did wreck and twist my pelvis.

The effects of the accident were devastating. Anything related to the pelvic area of my body was seriously impacted, including bowels and periods. I had been mad keen on sport, but that all stopped. For years, I struggled to work even part time and as time went on, my life became more and more limited.

Over time, I also started to suffer from chronic fatigue and was diagnosed with ME. I have a sensitivity to medication so tend to go down the alternative medicine route. Osteopathy and acupuncture helped enormously, but over a period of six years, the ME worsened. I had no social life and was unable to do things most people would take for granted like go for a walk, go out for a meal, go to the cinema, shopping or holidays.

In depth

I decided to try homeopathy. The first thing I noticed was that I was able to discuss medical issues in much more depth than I have ever with my own GPs. Over five sessions, my homeopath prescribed me several remedies and the effects of these have been astonishing.

Even with a chronic illness, there is a world of difference between feeling very unwell every day and having a sense of well-being. The Arnica put me in the latter category—I breathe better, my joints loosen, my diaphragm releases and I have more energy.

I feel much more in control, particularly with the knowledge that I don't have to take medication every day. The fact that the remedies don't have side effects is extremely reassuring.

It's very much an ongoing journey but exploring homeopathy has left me hopeful for the future. I don't how or why it works, but if you get the right remedy, it's miraculous!"

CHRONIC PAIN

Chronic pain refers to persistent pain that lasts for an extended period, typically longer than three months. It can be caused by various factors, such as injury, inflammation, nerve damage, or underlying health conditions. Managing chronic pain can be challenging, and conventional treatments often focus on symptom management. Homeopathy offers natural remedies that may help alleviate chronic pain and improve overall well-being. Here's a brief introduction to chronic pain and some commonly used homeopathic remedies.

Homeopathic helpers

Arnica montana: This remedy is often suggested for chronic pain resulting from injuries or trauma. It can help reduce pain, swelling, and bruising. Arnica is commonly used topically as an ointment or gel.

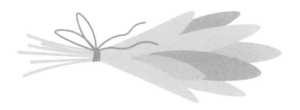

Rhus toxicodendron: Useful for chronic pain characterized by stiffness, aching, and aggravation on initial movement, which improves with continued motion. It is often recommended for pain associated with conditions like arthritis or fibromyalgia.

Hypericum perforatum: Indicated for chronic nerve pain, such as neuralgia or shooting, radiating pain. It can be helpful for pain following nerve injuries or surgeries.

Bryonia alba: This remedy is suitable for chronic pain with stitching or tearing sensations that worsen with movement. It can be beneficial for pain in joints, muscles, or organs, especially when worsened by exertion or touch.

Kali carbonicum: Useful for chronic pain, particularly in the back or joints, that is aggravated by cold and damp weather. It may be recommended for arthritic pain or spinal issues.

Coughs, Colds and Flu

Coughs, colds, and flu are common respiratory illnesses that can be caused by various viruses. They share some similar symptoms, but each condition has its distinct characteristics. Here's a brief introduction to these ailments and some homeopathic remedies that are commonly used to treat them:

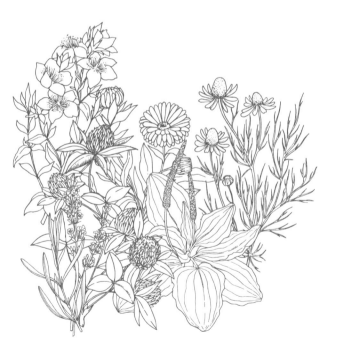

COUGHS

Coughs are reflex actions that help clear the airways of irritants, mucus, or foreign substances. They can be caused by viral infections, allergies, or irritants in the environment. Common types of coughs include dry coughs (non-productive) and productive coughs (with phlegm or mucus).

Homeopathic helpers

Drosera: Helpful for dry, spasmodic coughs that are worse at night or triggered by laughing or talking.

Bryonia: Indicated for dry, painful coughs that worsen with movement or deep breathing.

Hepar sulphuris: Useful for coughs with thick, yellow or green mucus that is difficult to expectorate.

Spongia tosta: Suitable for dry, barking coughs with a sensation of dryness and tightness in the throat.

COLDS

Colds are viral infections that primarily affect the nose and throat. They are characterized by symptoms such as a runny or congested nose, sneezing, sore throat, and mild coughing. Homeopathy can offer supportive care by addressing specific symptoms and promoting the body's natural healing response.

Homeopathic helpers

Aconite: Useful for colds that come on suddenly after exposure to cold wind or a fright. Symptoms may include fever, restlessness, and dry, croupy cough.

Allium cepa: Suggested for a cold with profuse, watery nasal discharge, along with burning and watering of the eyes.

Nux vomica: Helpful for colds caused by overexertion, excessive stress, or overindulgence in food or drink. Symptoms may include a stuffy nose, sneezing, and irritability.

Euphrasia: Suitable for colds with a profuse discharge of acrid, watery discharge from the eyes and nose.

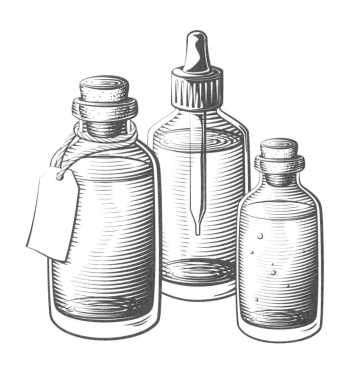

FLU

Flu is a viral infection caused by influenza viruses. It typically leads to more severe symptoms compared to a common cold. Symptoms may include high fever, body aches, fatigue, headache, sore throat, nasal congestion, and cough. Homeopathy can help by treating individual symptoms and boosting the body's immune response.

Homeopathic helpers

Gelsemium: Indicated for flu with heavy fatigue, weakness, chills, and aching muscles. It can be helpful during the early stages of the illness.

Bryonia: Useful for flu with body aches that worsen with movement, dry cough, and a desire to be left alone.

Eupatorium perfoliatum: Suitable for flu with intense body aches, bone pain, and fever. Thirst may be increased.

Oscillococcinum: A popular homeopathic remedy for flu, available in many countries as an over-the-counter product. It is used to relieve flu-like symptoms such as body aches, chills, and fatigue.

Cuts and grazes

Homeopathy can help aid cuts and grazes by promoting faster healing, reducing inflammation, and alleviating associated symptoms in minor cuts, but severe or deep wounds may require medical attention. These remedies are general suggestions, and the choice of remedy should be based on individual symptoms, the specific context of the cut or graze, and the person's overall health. It's advisable to consult with a qualified homeopath or healthcare professional for a proper evaluation and personalized recommendations based on your specific case. Additionally, it's important to clean the wound thoroughly, apply appropriate dressings or bandages, and follow basic wound care practices for optimal healing.

Homeopathic helpers

Calendula: Calendula is a well-known remedy for promoting wound healing. It can help reduce inflammation, prevent infection, and facilitate the regeneration of skin cells. Calendula ointment or cream can be applied topically to the affected area.

Staphysagria: This remedy is indicated for cuts or incisions that are slow to heal and tend to become easily infected. It can help promote healing, reduce pain, and prevent infection.

Hypericum: It is suitable for cuts or grazes that involve nerve-rich areas or injuries to the fingers, toes, or puncture wounds. Hypericum can help alleviate pain, reduce the risk of infection, and promote nerve healing.

Ledum palustre: This remedy is helpful for puncture wounds or cuts caused by sharp objects, such as nails or thorns. Ledum can help reduce swelling, prevent infection, and facilitate healing.

Silicea: It is indicated for cuts or wounds that are slow to heal, prone to infection, or have difficulty closing. Silicea can promote the expulsion of foreign objects, aid in the healing process, and strengthen the immune response.

CYSTITIS

The medical term for inflammation of the bladder, this irritating health issue is typically caused by a bacterial infection but can also be triggered by irritants and certain medications. It is more common in women than in men and can cause symptoms such as frequent urination, a strong urge to urinate, pain or discomfort in the lower abdomen, and a burning sensation during urination.

Homeopathy can help by addressing the underlying causes, reducing inflammation, and relieving associated symptoms, but seek medical attention if symptoms persist or worsen, as antibiotics may be necessary to treat bacterial cystitis and prevent complications.

Homeopathic helpers

Cantharis: This remedy is often recommended for intense burning and cutting pain during urination. The person may have a strong urge to urinate but pass only small amounts of urine.

Apis mellifica: It is suitable for cystitis accompanied by a stinging or burning sensation during urination. The person may experience frequent, urgent urination, but passing urine provides only temporary relief.

Staphysagria: This remedy is used for cystitis that develops after sexual intercourse. The person may experience a constant urge to urinate, but passing urine can be difficult and unsatisfying. The condition may be associated with feelings of anger or resentment.

Pulsatilla: It is indicated for cystitis with a sensation of pressure in the bladder, and the person may have to urinate frequently, especially at night. The urine may be scanty and pale. Pulsatilla is often recommended for cases associated with mild, weepy, or changeable emotional states.

Sarsaparilla: This remedy is helpful for cystitis with severe burning pain at the end of urination. The person may have to strain to pass urine, and the pain may extend from the bladder to the urethra.

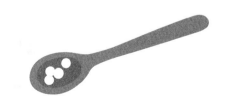

DENTAL HEALTH

Dental issues encompass a wide range of conditions affecting the teeth, gums, and oral cavity. Common dental problems include toothache, tooth decay, gum disease (gingivitis or periodontitis), oral thrush, and dental abscesses. While proper dental hygiene and regular dental check-ups with a qualified practitioner are essential for maintaining oral health, homeopathy can be used as a complementary approach to support the body's natural healing processes and alleviate symptoms.

Homeopathic helpers

Plantago: This remedy is often indicated for toothache with sharp, shooting pains that extend to the face or ears. The pain may worsen from cold drinks and touch but improve from biting on the affected tooth.

Arnica: Useful for dental pain or soreness following dental procedures or trauma. It can help reduce swelling, bruising, and alleviate discomfort.

Mercurius solubilis: Indicated for gum inflammation, bleeding gums, and painful, loose teeth. The person may experience increased salivation with a metallic taste in the mouth.

Hepar sulphuris: Helpful for dental abscesses with throbbing, stitching pain, and sensitivity to touch or cold. The person may have bad breath and swollen, tender gums.

Kreosotum: Indicated for tooth decay with rapidly progressing cavities, dark or discoloured teeth, and increased sensitivity to cold drinks.

Silicea: Suitable for dental problems associated with brittle teeth, gum abscesses, and slow healing of oral wounds. It can also help expel foreign objects lodged between teeth or gums.

Calcarea fluorica: Useful for strengthening tooth enamel, preventing cavities, and treating dental caries.

Staphysagria: Indicated for tooth pain resulting from dental procedures or surgeries. It can help reduce postoperative pain and promote healing.

DEPRESSION

Depression is a complex mental health condition that can be caused by various factors, including biological, genetic, environmental, and psychological factors. While homeopathy cannot cure this condition, it can address the underlying causes of depression and support overall well-being. It approaches depression holistically, taking into account the physical, mental, and emotional aspects and remedies are selected based on your unique symptom picture and overall health. If you or someone you know is experiencing depression, it's essential to seek help from a qualified healthcare professional who can provide a comprehensive assessment and develop a suitable treatment plan.

Homeopathic helpers

Ignatia amara: This remedy is often used for acute grief or emotional distress, especially after the loss of a loved one. It can help with symptoms of sadness, mood swings, and a tendency to suppress emotions.

Natrum muriaticum: When there is a history of suppressed emotions or grief, and the person tends to isolate themselves, Natrum muriaticum may be considered. It can address feelings of sadness, loneliness, and a desire for solitude.

Aurum metallicum: This remedy is commonly used for depression with a sense of deep hopelessness, worthlessness, and thoughts of self-harm. It may be helpful when depression is associated with work-related stress or a sense of failure.

Arsenicum album: When there is anxiety along with depression, and the person is restless and fearful, Arsenicum album may be indicated. It can help with feelings of restlessness and agitation.

Sepia: This remedy is often used for depression in women, especially during or after menopause. It can address feelings of indifference, irritability, and mood swings.

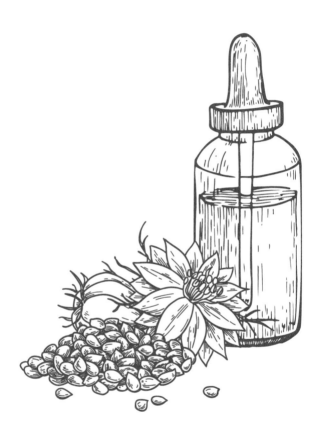

CASE STUDY

Lindsey's story

**A chance encounter with a homeopath
changed the course of Lindsey's life**

"In 2012, I was living in Spain when I had
my first baby. It was a difficult birth and
the whole experience was quite traumatic.
I ended up having a c-section, but my
husband wasn't allowed into the room and
I didn't speak the language. It felt as though
lots of invasive things were happening to
me that I didn't understand.

Afterwards, I started to suffer from
low mood, anxiety and painful hips. My
throat felt tight all the time, like I couldn't
breathe. All of which was exacerbated by
the usual early motherhood issues like sleep
deprivation.

I slowly started to heal

As luck would have it, I had befriended a neighbour whose husband was a renowned homeopath. He would charge patients at his private clinic but also treat people in need for free in his hometown. Once I started seeing him, it was like peeling an onion. Together we uncovered some longstanding emotional issues and I slowly started to heal.

Then I fell pregnant again and because of my previous experience, I started to feel extremely anxious. I persuaded my husband to move back to the UK and my son was born there. At first, everything seemed better but then the anxiety and throat tightening started again.

I was at home with a two-year-old and a baby, with virtually no support. I did investigate homeopathic treatment, but it was just too expensive. When I went to my GP, I felt as though he didn't really understand. He prescribed betablockers, even though I was breastfeeding.

I muddled along for several years, but what with covid and my husband and I both being made redundant, the stress of the previous years had really taken their toll. I felt incredibly low and had no joy in my life. The future didn't hold anything interesting for me and I felt trapped and overwhelmed by a sense of responsibility. At the same time, I was experiencing pain in my neck and hip."

I feel better than I have for years

I knew from previous experience that my GP would only offer me anti-depressants and beta blockers and I really wanted to go down the homeopathic route. Money was still tight so I didn't think it would be an option, but then my mum told me about a charitable clinic in Liverpool that offered very low-cost care, so I made an appointment with a practitioner who prescribed a host of remedies to tackle my various symptoms, including Sepia, Nat mur and Calc carb. Fast forward to the present day and I feel better than I have for 20 years. My life is back on track and I am happy and optimistic for the future. My sessions with Emma were undoubtedly key to this. There was a moment where things started to change and I began to feel differently. It's a gentle transformation but it really gets to the root of the problem.

By tackling the underlying emotions, as well as my physical symptoms, I've been able to achieve a sense of well-being that I never thought possible. Homeopathy may be gentle but it's enormously powerful too."

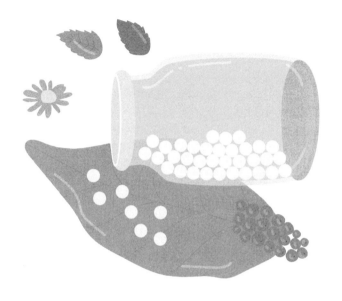

DIGESTIVE HEALTH

Digestive issues encompass a range of conditions that affect the digestive system, including the stomach, intestines, and other related organs. Common digestive problems include indigestion, acid reflux, bloating, gas, constipation, diarrhoea, and irritable bowel syndrome (IBS). While lifestyle changes, dietary modifications, and medical advice are often necessary, homeopathic remedies can be used to support the body's natural healing processes and provide relief from digestive discomfort. Additionally, maintaining a balanced diet, drinking plenty of water, and practicing good eating habits can contribute to optimal digestive health.

Homeopathic helpers

Nux vomica: This remedy is often indicated for digestive issues related to overindulgence in food, alcohol, or stimulants. It can help alleviate symptoms such as indigestion, heartburn, bloating, and constipation.

Arsenicum album: Useful for digestive problems accompanied by anxiety, restlessness, and a desire for small sips of water. It can help relieve symptoms of food poisoning, diarrhoea, and vomiting.

Lycopodium: Indicated for digestive issues such as bloating, gas, and indigestion that worsen in the late afternoon or evening. The person may experience a sensation of fullness after eating a small amount of food.

Carbo vegetabilis: Helpful for digestive problems accompanied by excessive gas, bloating, and belching. It can also relieve symptoms of heartburn and indigestion.

Pulsatilla: Suitable for digestive issues that arise from rich, fatty foods or a change in diet. It can help relieve symptoms such as bloating, indigestion, and loose stools.

Lachesis: Indicated for digestive issues accompanied by a feeling of constriction or tightness in the abdomen. It can help alleviate symptoms of indigestion, acid reflux, and constipation.

Podophyllum: Useful for digestive problems with profuse, watery diarrhoea and gurgling in the abdomen. It can also help relieve symptoms of colic in infants.

Sulphur: Indicated for various digestive issues, including diarrhoea, constipation, and bloating. The person may experience burning sensations in the stomach or rectum.

EARACHE

Earache refers to pain or discomfort in the ear, which can vary in intensity and may be accompanied by other symptoms such as ear fullness, hearing loss, or fever. There are several potential causes of earaches, including ear infection in the middle ear, known as otitis media which can be bacterial or viral in nature and often occurs in children. Other causes of earache are earwax build up, which can put pressure on the ear drum, and swimmers' ear, or external otitis, which is an infection of the outer ear canal typically caused by exposure to water, leading to ear pain and inflammation.

Homeopathy can offer supportive treatment for earaches by addressing the underlying causes and providing relief from symptoms. Remember, seeking medical attention is crucial for severe or persistent ear pain, particularly in cases involving young children or complications such as high fever or hearing loss.

Homeopathic helpers

Belladonna: Often indicated for sudden, intense ear pain that comes on rapidly. The ear may be red, hot, and throbbing. It is typically used for acute ear infections.

Pulsatilla: Useful for earaches with a sensation of pressure or fullness in the ear. The pain is often worse at night or in a warm room. Pulsatilla is commonly prescribed for earaches associated with colds or after exposure to wind.

Chamomilla: Suitable for earaches accompanied by extreme irritability and restlessness, particularly in children. The pain may be sharp, and warmth or rocking can bring some relief.

Hepar sulphuris: It is indicated for earaches that are very sensitive to touch and accompanied by offensive-smelling discharge. The pain may be throbbing, and the person may be irritable and chilly.

Silicea: Often used for chronic or recurrent ear infections. It can be helpful when there are discharge and pressure in the ear, and the person feels chilly and lacks confidence.

ECZEMA

Also known as atopic dermatitis, this is a chronic skin condition characterised by inflamed, itchy, and dry patches of skin. While eczema is a complex condition that requires professional guidance, homeopathy can offer natural remedies that might help alleviate symptoms and support overall skin health. Remember, these remedies are just a starting point, and it's important to consult with a qualified homeopath for a thorough evaluation of your symptoms and to receive personalized treatment. Additionally, natural skincare, avoiding triggers and maintaining a healthy lifestyle can contribute to managing eczema effectively.

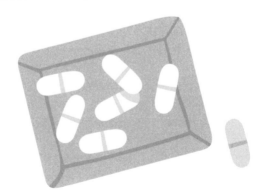

Homeopathic helpers

Graphites: This remedy is often indicated for dry, rough, and itchy eczema with thickened and oozing skin. The affected areas may be worse at night and may crack or bleed easily. Graphites can be beneficial for eczema that tends to be worse in cold weather.

Sulphur: Useful for red, itchy, and burning eczema with a tendency to worsen with heat. The affected skin may be dry, rough, and appear dirty. Sulphur is often prescribed for individuals who are warm-blooded and tend to perspire.

Mezereum: Indicated for eczema with intense itching, burning, and formation of thick crusts or scabs. The affected areas may ooze a sticky fluid, and scratching can lead to bleeding and thickening of the skin.

Rhus toxicodendron: This remedy is helpful for eczema with intense itching, especially when the itching is relieved by applying heat or warm water. The affected skin may be red, swollen, and have a blistered appearance.

Natrum muriaticum: Suitable for eczema that appears in the bends of joints, such as elbows and knees, or around the hairline. The skin may be dry, itchy, and cracked, and exposure to sunlight may worsen the condition. Individuals needing Natrum muriaticum may have a history of grief or emotional sensitivity.

Apis mellifica: Indicated for eczema with redness, swelling, and intense itching that is relieved by cold applications. The affected skin may have a puffy appearance and feel hot to the touch.

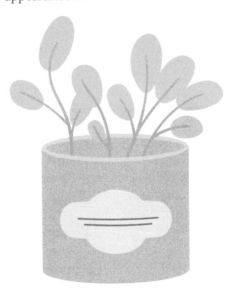

ENDOMETRIOSIS

Endometriosis is a chronic condition where tissue similar to the lining of the uterus (endometrium) grows outside the uterus, commonly affecting the ovaries, fallopian tubes, and pelvic tissues. It can cause symptoms such as pelvic pain, painful periods, heavy menstrual bleeding, infertility, and gastrointestinal issues. While homeopathy cannot cure endometriosis (and remember it is important to consult a medical professional for treatment), it may offer support in managing symptoms and promoting overall well-being.

Homeopathic helpers

Sepia: This remedy is often indicated for women with endometriosis who experience heavy and painful periods, along with a sense of bearing down or dragging sensation in the pelvis. There may be associated mood swings, irritability, and fatigue.

Lachesis: Useful for intense and burning pelvic pain, especially before and during periods. The pain may worsen with pressure or tight clothing, and there may be a sensation of constriction or suffocation.

Platina: This is indicated for severe pain during intercourse (dyspareunia) or for those who have a heightened sexual drive. There may be a sense of dryness and sensitivity in the vaginal area.

Belladonna: This remedy may be helpful during acute flare-ups of endometriosis, especially when there is sudden and intense pelvic pain that comes and goes. The pain may be accompanied by a flushed face, throbbing headache, and high fever.

Nux vomica: Suitable for digestive issues triggered by endometriosis such as constipation, bloating, and abdominal discomfort. These symptoms may be aggravated by stress, sedentary lifestyle, and dietary indiscretions.

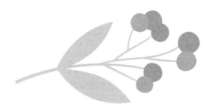

FATIGUE

Do you suffer from feeling of tiredness, lack of energy and decreased motivation? Homeopathic remedies can help to stimulate the body's inherent healing abilities, address the underlying imbalances, and restore vitality. Additionally, lifestyle factors such as getting adequate rest, maintaining a balanced diet, managing stress, and incorporating regular exercise can also contribute to improving energy levels and combating fatigue.

Homeopathic helpers

Gelsemium: This remedy is often indicated for fatigue accompanied by heaviness and weakness in the limbs, a desire to be left alone, and a lack of motivation. It is particularly useful when fatigue is associated with anticipation, performance anxiety, or stage fright.

Arnica: When fatigue is the result of physical exertion, overexertion, or trauma, Arnica may be helpful. It can assist in reducing muscle soreness, promoting recovery, and relieving mental and physical exhaustion.

Nux vomica: This remedy is indicated when fatigue is associated with a sedentary lifestyle, excessive work, irregular sleep patterns, and overindulgence in stimulants like coffee or alcohol. It can help restore balance and improve overall energy levels.

Kali phosphoricum: When fatigue is accompanied by mental exhaustion, irritability, and feeling overwhelmed, Kali phosphoricum may be considered. It can support mental clarity, relieve stress, and improve energy levels.

Ginkgo biloba: As mentioned earlier, Ginkgo biloba can be used as a homeopathic remedy for general fatigue. It is believed to enhance blood circulation, especially to the brain, which may help improve cognitive function, concentration, and overall vitality.

FEVER

Fever is a natural response of the body to various underlying causes, typically indicating an immune response to an infection or inflammation. It is often a sign that the body is fighting off an illness. Common causes of fever include viral or bacterial infections, such as the flu, common cold, urinary tract or respiratory infections, certain inflammatory diseases, like rheumatoid arthritis or inflammatory bowel disease and the side effects of medications or vaccines. Homeopathy can help manage fever by supporting the body's natural healing mechanisms and addressing the underlying causes. Additionally, staying well-hydrated, getting adequate rest, and using appropriate measures to manage body temperature, such as tepid sponging can help.

Homeopathic helpers

Belladonna: This remedy is often indicated for sudden, intense fevers with hot, red skin. The person may experience throbbing headaches, dilated pupils, and have a dry mouth. The fever may come on rapidly and be accompanied by restlessness.

Aconitum napellus: It is suitable for fevers that occur suddenly, often after exposure to cold, dry winds. The person may feel restless, anxious, and have a rapid pulse. The skin may feel hot and dry.

Ferrum phosphoricum: This remedy is indicated for fevers that are mild to moderate in intensity. The person may have a flushed face, feel weak or fatigued, and experience a slight increase in temperature. It is often used during the early stages of a fever.

Gelsemium: It is helpful for fevers accompanied by weakness, fatigue, and chills. The person may have a headache, heavy eyelids, and feel drowsy or sluggish. The fever may be gradual in onset.

Bryonia: This remedy is indicated for fevers accompanied by intense thirst and dryness of the mucous membranes. The person may experience worsening of symptoms with movement and prefer to remain still. The fever may be associated with body aches.

FIBROMYALGIA

This is a chronic condition characterised by widespread musculoskeletal pain, fatigue, sleep disturbances, and cognitive difficulties. It is a complex disorder with no known cure, and the treatment primarily focuses on managing symptoms and improving quality of life. While homeopathy cannot directly treat fibromyalgia, it can support overall health and well-being and help manage certain symptoms. Additionally, lifestyle modifications, stress management techniques, gentle exercise, and a healthy diet can also play a role in managing fibromyalgia symptoms effectively.

Homeopathic helpers

Rhus toxicodendron: This remedy is often indicated for people experiencing stiffness, aching and restless discomfort that worsens with rest and improves with movement. They may have difficulty getting out of bed in the morning due to stiffness and may experience relief from warm applications.

Bryonia alba: Useful for fibromyalgia characterised by intense, stitching, and tearing pain that worsens with movement and is relieved by rest. The person may feel better with pressure applied to the affected areas and may experience aggravation in cold weather.

Arnica montana: Indicated for soreness, bruised sensations, and a feeling as if the body has been beaten. The pain may be worse with touch or pressure, and there may be a general feeling of fatigue.

Ruta graveolens: This remedy is suitable for stiffness and pain in the muscles and joints, like that experienced after excessive physical exertion. The pain may be worse with cold and dampness and may feel better with gentle motion and warmth.

Kali phosphoricum: Useful for people who experience mental and physical exhaustion, weakness, and a lack of energy. They may also have difficulty concentrating and experience mood swings.

FOOD POISONING

Food poisoning is an illness caused by consuming contaminated food or water. It occurs when harmful bacteria, viruses, parasites, or toxins present in the food enter the body and cause infection or toxin-mediated reactions. Common symptoms of food poisoning include nausea, vomiting, diarrhoea, abdominal pain, fever, and sometimes, dehydration.

Homeopathy can be helpful in addressing the symptoms and promoting recovery from food poisoning. However, it's important to note that severe cases of food poisoning may require medical attention, especially if symptoms are persistent or severe.

Homeopathic helpers

Arsenicum album: This remedy is often indicated for food poisoning with symptoms of vomiting and diarrhoea. The person may experience intense anxiety, restlessness, and a desire for small sips of water. Symptoms are typically worse at night and improve with warmth.

Nux vomica: It is suitable for food poisoning with symptoms such as nausea, vomiting, and indigestion. The person may feel irritable, impatient, and have a desire for spicy or stimulant foods. Symptoms are often worse in the morning or after eating.

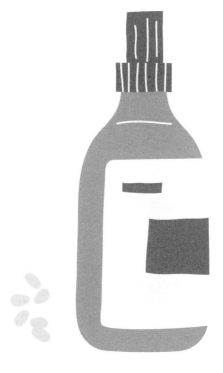

Veratrum album: This remedy is used for food poisoning with profuse vomiting and diarrhoea. The person may have cold sweats, extreme weakness, and a desire for ice-cold drinks. Symptoms may be accompanied by cramps and a pale face.

Podophyllum: It is indicated for food poisoning with profuse, gushing diarrhoea. The stool may be watery, offensive-smelling, and may occur early in the morning. The person may experience weakness and abdominal pain.

Phosphorus: This remedy is helpful for food poisoning with symptoms such as vomiting, diarrhoea, and weakness. The person may have a strong thirst for cold drinks and feel anxious or fearful.

HAEMORRHOIDS

Also known as piles, these are swollen veins in the rectum or anus that can cause discomfort, pain, itching, and sometimes bleeding. They are caused by various factors including straining during bowel movements, chronic diarrhoea, pregnancy and obesity.

Homeopathy can help relieve symptoms associated with haemorrhoids and address underlying factors contributing to their development. Additionally, maintaining good bowel habits, avoiding excessive straining, and incorporating dietary changes to promote regular bowel movements can complement homeopathic treatment for haemorrhoids.

Homeopathic helpers

Aesculus hippocastanum: This remedy is indicated for haemorrhoids with backache and a feeling of fullness or heaviness in the rectum. The haemorrhoids may be large, swollen, and painful.

Hamamelis virginiana: It is suitable for haemorrhoids with bleeding and a feeling of rawness or soreness in the rectal area. The bleeding is often dark in colour.

Collinsonia canadensis: This remedy is used for haemorrhoids with a sensation of constriction or as if there is a stick lodged in the rectum. There may be constipation with hard, dry stools.

Nux vomica: It is indicated for haemorrhoids caused by excessive straining during bowel movements, especially due to a sedentary lifestyle or overindulgence in stimulants like alcohol or coffee.

Sulphur: This remedy is helpful for haemorrhoids that are itchy, burning, and accompanied by a feeling of heat in the anus. There may be a tendency for constipation alternating with diarrhoea.

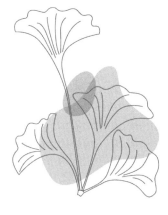

HAY FEVER

Hay fever, also known as allergic rhinitis, is an allergic reaction to airborne substances such as pollen, dust mites, or pet dander. It typically manifests as symptoms like sneezing, itching, runny nose, nasal congestion, and watery eyes. While conventional treatments such as antihistamines and nasal sprays are commonly used, homeopathy offers natural remedies that may help alleviate hay fever symptoms. Homeopathic treatment aims to address the underlying imbalances and strengthen the body's natural defences against allergens. In addition to homeopathic remedies, allergen avoidance, maintaining a clean indoor environment, using nasal saline rinses, and wearing sunglasses can also help manage hay fever symptoms effectively.

Homeopathic helpers

Allium cepa: This remedy is often indicated for hay fever with profuse watery discharge from the nose, along with sneezing and burning sensation in the eyes. The person may feel better in open air and worse in a warm room.

Natrum muriaticum: Useful for hay fever with sneezing, watery discharge from the nose, and a sensation of a tickling or crawling in the nose. The person may experience relief near the seashore or during perspiration.

Sabadilla: Indicated for hay fever with violent sneezing, itching, and watery discharge from the nose. The eyes may be red and watering, and there may be a sensation of a lump in the throat.

Euphrasia: This remedy is suitable for hay fever with profuse watery discharge from the eyes, along with burning and redness. The nose may also be watery, and symptoms may worsen in the open air and sunlight.

Arsenicum album: Useful for hay fever with a burning sensation in the nose and eyes, along with a thin, watery discharge. The person may experience restlessness and anxiety and feel better with warm drinks.

HEART HEALTH

Heart complaints encompass a range of conditions affecting the heart, including cardiovascular diseases, such as hypertension, angina, arrhythmias, and heart failure. While homeopathy cannot directly treat serious heart conditions, it can support overall cardiovascular health and help manage certain symptoms. Remember homeopathic treatment for heart conditions should always be used in conjunction with conventional medical care. Homeopathy can support overall well-being, alleviate certain symptoms, and promote a sense of balance. However, it should never replace or delay proper medical diagnosis and treatment. If you or someone you know is experiencing heart-related symptoms, it is crucial to seek immediate medical attention and follow the guidance of a qualified healthcare professional.

Homeopathic helpers

Crataegus oxyacantha: This remedy is often indicated for heart complaints, especially when there is weakness, fatigue, and a sensation of pressure or tightness in the chest. It can be used as a supportive remedy for heart conditions.

Digitalis purpurea: Useful for heart complaints with symptoms of irregular or slow heartbeat, palpitations, and fainting. It may be considered in cases of heart failure or arrhythmias.

Cactus grandiflorus: Indicated for heart complaints with a feeling of constriction or tightness in the chest, as if gripped by an iron band. It can be helpful for angina and certain types of heart palpitations.

Aurum metallicum: This remedy is suitable for heart complaints associated with emotional stress, depression, and a sense of heaviness or pressure in the chest. It may be considered for individuals with a history of heart disease or hypertension.

Kalmia latifolia: Useful for heart complaints with sharp, burning, shooting and stabbing pains that radiate to the scapula and arm. It can be considered for angina and heart conditions affecting the left side of the chest.

HIGH BLOOD PRESSURE

While homeopathy can't treat high blood pressure (or hypertension) itself, it can offer supportive care by addressing your overall health, stress levels and specific symptoms related to high blood pressure. Remember that homeopathy should always be used in conjunction with appropriate medical supervision, especially for conditions like hypertension that require careful management to prevent complications.

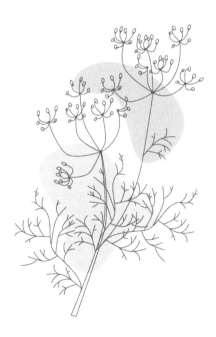

Homeopathic helpers

Nux vomica: For hypertension due to stress, sedentary lifestyle, and excess consumption of stimulants like coffee and spicy foods.

Lycopodium: For people with high blood pressure and digestive issues or a tendency to overeat.

Glonoinum: For hypertension with severe headaches and a sensation of fullness in the head.

Crataegus: For individuals with hypertension and heart-related symptoms like palpitations or a weak heart.

Rauwolfia serpentina: This remedy is sometimes used in combination with conventional antihypertensive drugs to support blood pressure management.

INDIGESTION

Indigestion, also known as dyspepsia, refers to a condition characterized by discomfort or pain in the upper abdomen. It is commonly associated with symptoms such as bloating, belching, nausea, heartburn, and a feeling of fullness or early satiety. Indigestion can be caused by various factors, including overeating, spicy or fatty foods, stress and anxiety or chronic acid reflux, where stomach acid flows back into the oesophagus. Homeopathy

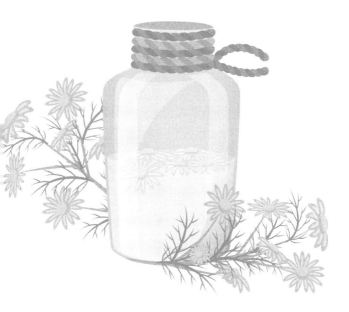

can help alleviate symptoms of indigestion and address underlying imbalances in the digestive system but it's advisable to consult with a qualified homeopath or healthcare professional for a proper evaluation.

Homeopathic helpers

Nux vomica: This remedy is often indicated for indigestion due to overeating, alcohol consumption, or spicy foods. The person may experience a sensation of heaviness or pressure in the stomach, along with nausea, heartburn, and a desire for stimulants like coffee or alcohol.

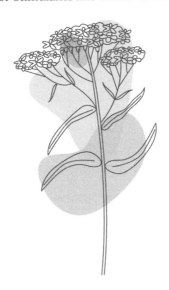

Pulsatilla: It is suitable for indigestion accompanied by a feeling of fullness and bloating after eating. The person may experience belching, a lack of thirst, and a preference for rich or fatty foods. Symptoms are often relieved by gentle exercise and fresh air.

Carbo vegetabilis: This remedy is used for indigestion with bloating, flatulence, and a sense of heaviness in the abdomen. The person may feel chilly, weak, and have a craving for fresh air.

Lycopodium: It is indicated for indigestion characterized by bloating, gas, and a sensation of fullness after eating a small amount. The person may have an excessive appetite but feel satisfied quickly. Symptoms often worsen in the late afternoon or evening.

Natrum phosphoricum: This remedy is helpful for indigestion with sour belching and heartburn. The person may experience acid regurgitation and a sour taste in the mouth.

IBS

Irritable Bowel Syndrome (IBS) is a chronic gastrointestinal disorder characterised by abdominal pain, bloating, changes in bowel habits (such as diarrhoea or constipation), and discomfort. While the exact cause of IBS is unknown, it is believed to involve a combination of factors, including abnormal gut motility, hypersensitivity to certain foods, stress, and changes in the gut microbiota. Homeopathy offers natural remedies that may help alleviate IBS symptoms and promote digestive balance. Additionally, dietary modifications, stress management techniques, regular exercise, and maintaining a healthy lifestyle can play a significant role in managing symptoms effectively.

Homeopathic helpers

Nux vomica: This remedy is often indicated for individuals with IBS who experience bloating, abdominal pain, and a constant urge to have a bowel movement. Symptoms may worsen after eating, with a tendency toward constipation.

Lycopodium: Useful for IBS with bloating, gas, and a sensation of fullness in the abdomen. There may be rumbling sounds in the abdomen and a tendency toward constipation.

Pulsatilla: Indicated for individuals with IBS who experience alternating diarrhoea and constipation. Symptoms may be triggered or worsened by consuming rich or fatty foods, and there may be a craving for sweets.

China officinalis: This remedy is suitable for individuals with IBS who experience abdominal pain and bloating, along with diarrhoea or loose stools. Symptoms may be accompanied by weakness, fatigue, and anaemia.

Argentum nitricum: Useful for individuals with IBS who experience bloating, flatulence, and explosive diarrhoea. Symptoms may be worsened by anxiety and anticipation.

INDIGESTION

Also known as dyspepsia, this common health complaint has a range of symptoms that occur in the upper abdomen, including discomfort, pain, bloating, and a feeling of fullness after eating. It can be caused by various factors such as overeating, eating too quickly, fatty or spicy foods, stress, or certain medical conditions. While homeopathy can help to relieve the symptoms, lifestyle modifications such as eating smaller meals, avoiding trigger foods, practicing mindful eating, managing stress, and maintaining a healthy weight can also support digestive health.

Homeopathic helpers

Nux vomica: This remedy is often indicated for indigestion caused by overeating, excessive alcohol consumption, or a sedentary lifestyle. Symptoms may include heartburn, acid reflux, bloating, and a feeling of fullness. There may also be irritability, impatience, and sensitivity to noise.

Carbo vegetabilis: This remedy is useful for indigestion with bloating and distention of the abdomen. There may be a sensation of heaviness or pressure in the stomach, with belching and flatulence providing temporary relief. The person may feel weak, chilly, and have a desire for fresh air.

Pulsatilla: Indigestion that worsens after eating rich, fatty, or creamy foods and is accompanied by bloating, burping, and a sense of heaviness may respond well to Pulsatilla. The person may have a changeable appetite, craving for comforting foods, and a tendency to be weepy or emotionally sensitive.

Lycopodium: This remedy is often indicated for indigestion with bloating and a sense of fullness after eating a small amount of food. Symptoms may include belching, flatulence, and a tendency towards constipation. The person may have a lack of self-confidence and fear of public speaking.

Natrum phosphoricum: This remedy can be beneficial for indigestion with an excessive amount of acid, leading to sour belching, heartburn, and a heavy sensation in the stomach. The person may prefer acidic foods, such as citrus fruits, and may experience bloating and flatulence.

INFERTILITY

Homeopathic remedies can be used to support fertility by addressing underlying imbalances and promoting overall well-being, but fertility issues can have numerous causes so individualized treatment really is key. You should always consult with a qualified homeopath for a comprehensive assessment and personalized treatment plan and to work in conjunction with conventional medical care, as there may be underlying medical factors that require attention.

Homeopathic helpers

Sepia: This remedy is often indicated for hormonal imbalances and irregular menstrual cycles. It may be useful for women experiencing decreased libido, heavy or prolonged periods, or symptoms related to hormonal changes.

Pulsatilla: This remedy is often suited for women with irregular or suppressed menstrual cycles, emotional sensitivity, and a tendency to weep easily. It may be helpful for addressing hormonal imbalances and promoting regular ovulation.

Sabina: This remedy is often used for women with a history of recurrent miscarriages or heavy bleeding during periods. It may help address issues related to implantation and promote a healthy pregnancy.

Lycopodium: This remedy is often indicated for men with low sperm count, erectile dysfunction, or premature ejaculation. It may help improve sperm quality and promote overall reproductive health.

Natrum muriaticum: This remedy is often used for women with irregular menstrual cycles, especially if associated with grief, suppressed emotions, or a history of contraceptive use. It may help restore hormonal balance and support fertility.

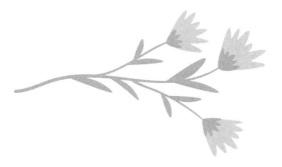

INSOMNIA

Sleep issues can encompass a variety of conditions, including insomnia, difficulty falling asleep, staying asleep or experiencing restful sleep. Sleep disturbances can have various causes, such as stress, anxiety, physical discomfort or lifestyle factors. Homeopathy offers a holistic approach to addressing sleep issues by considering your unique symptoms and overall well-being. Additionally, establishing a relaxing bedtime routine, maintaining a comfortable sleep environment, and practicing good sleep hygiene can contribute to improved sleep quality.

Homeopathic helpers

Coffea cruda: This remedy is indicated for sleeplessness due to an overactive mind, racing thoughts, and excessive mental stimulation. It can help calm the mind and promote restful sleep.

Nux vomica: Useful for sleep disruptions caused by stress, overwork, or a sedentary lifestyle. It is beneficial for individuals who wake up feeling unrefreshed or have trouble falling back asleep after waking up during the night.

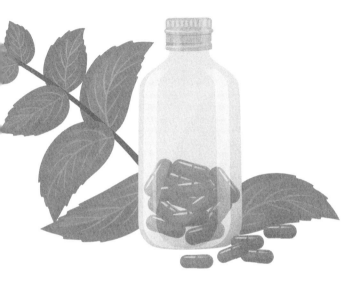

Passiflora incarnata: Indicated for difficulty falling asleep due to an overactive mind and restlessness. It can help promote relaxation and ease into sleep.

Arsenicum album: Helpful for sleep issues associated with anxiety, restlessness, and a sense of unease. It is particularly suitable for individuals who wake up in the night and can't get back to sleep.

Pulsatilla: Indicated for sleep disturbances due to emotional sensitivity, weepiness, and frequent changes in mood. It can be beneficial for individuals who feel better when comforted and may experience sleep disruptions from minor disturbances.

Lycopodium: Useful for sleep issues associated with digestive disturbances, such as bloating and gas. It can help improve sleep quality by addressing underlying digestive imbalances.

Chamomilla: Indicated for sleep problems in infants and children, particularly when they are restless, irritable, and have difficulty calming down. It can also be helpful for teething-related sleep disruptions.

Ignatia amara: Suitable for sleep disturbances due to grief, emotional distress, or recent loss. It can help promote emotional healing and support restful sleep.

CASE STUDY

Melissa's story

Melissa used homeopathy to help her recover from early menopause—and changed her life in the process

In early 2013, I was feeling at a very low ebb but put it down to the fact I had two small children. I had only just stopped breastfeeding and of course wasn't getting much sleep! I had also been diagnosed with a Vitamin D deficiency.

In June, I discovered a pea-sized lump on my right breast. I had lost my mum 18 months before to ovarian cancer and discovered that I carried the BRCA1 gene. Because of this, I was fast-tracked for an NHS mammogram, which revealed I had a stage 1 grade 3 tumour.

In August, I underwent a double mastectomy, followed by six months of horrendous chemotherapy. I felt absolutely terrible and had no energy. I was still grieving my mum; my eldest child was starting school and I couldn't even pick up my eighteen-month-old. On top of that, we moved to a new house—it really was a very bad time for our family.

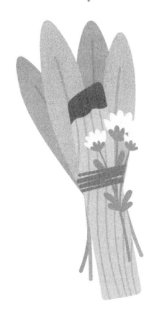

Suffering terrible menopause symptoms

By Easter of the following year, I was starting to recover. My hair was growing back and I was able to do school runs again. But because of the BRCA1 gene, I opted to have an oopherectomy (removal of ovaries and fallopian tubes) which led to a medically-induced menopause at the age of 35.

With a natural menopause, your body has time to adjust during the perimenopause period. But I was straight into it, suffering with terrible symptoms—joint pain, complete exhaustion and night sweats. My GP had prescribed me an effective—but very brutal—anti-depressant to tackle these and for a time, the medication worked. But when I tried to wean myself off it, the symptoms returned worse than before. I couldn't see a way out.

My life has changed in so many ways

Then a homeopath prescribed several remedies and herbal tonics, as well as providing some excellent dietary and lifestyle advice. I noticed a gradual improvement from the outset and after six months, I was off the medication and symptom-free.

I was so impressed with the whole homeopathic approach that in I attended a weekend course with a view to becoming a homeopath myself. At the end of the weekend, I was hooked! I am now in my fourth and final year of learning and practicing under supervision.

Having breast cancer and early menopause could have been an entirely negative experience. But those experiences have led to me where I am today so for that I am enormously grateful. My previous role as an Ofsted inspector feels a very long way off!"

MENOPAUSE

Menopause is a natural phase in a woman's life when her menstrual cycles cease, typically occurring between the ages of 45 and 55. It is associated with hormonal changes, particularly a decline in oestrogen levels, which can lead to a variety of symptoms. Common menopausal symptoms include hot flushes, night sweats, mood swings, sleep disturbances, vaginal dryness, and changes in libido. It's important to remember that homeopathic treatment is individualized, so for best results you should consult a qualified homeopath who can assess your specific symptoms, overall health, and emotional state. Additionally, lifestyle modifications such as regular exercise, a balanced diet, stress management techniques, and getting enough rest can also contribute to a smoother menopausal transition and overall well-being.

Homeopathic helpers

Sepia: This remedy is often indicated for menopausal symptoms, such as hot flashes, irritability, and mood swings. There may be a feeling of heaviness in the pelvic area, and symptoms can improve with vigorous exercise.

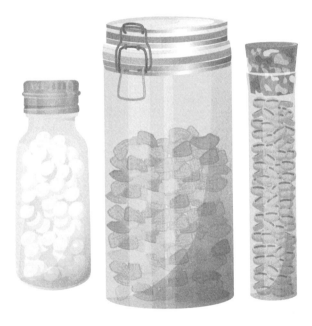

Lachesis: Useful for menopausal symptoms with intense hot flashes, especially on the left side of the body. There may be palpitations, mood swings, and a sense of being suffocated by tight clothing.

Pulsatilla: Indicated for menopausal symptoms accompanied by mood swings, weepiness, and a desire for consolation. Hot flashes may be accompanied by chills, and symptoms can improve with fresh air and gentle exercise.

Sanguinaria canadensis: This remedy is suitable for menopausal symptoms, particularly intense hot flashes and night sweats that begin on the face and spread upward. There may be headaches and a flushed face.

Ignatia amara: Useful for menopausal symptoms associated with emotional sensitivity, mood swings, and a tendency to suppress emotions. There may be sighing, difficulty sleeping, and a sensation of a lump in the throat.

MIGRAINES

Severe headaches that can cause intense throbbing or pulsating pain, they are often accompanied by other symptoms such as nausea, vomiting, sensitivity to light and sound, and visual disturbances. Migraines can significantly impact daily life and require a comprehensive approach for management. While consultation with a medical practitioner is essential, homeopathic remedies can help to provide relief during migraine attacks and may also address underlying imbalances to reduce the frequency and intensity of migraines over time. Lifestyle modifications, stress management, and identifying and avoiding triggers are also important aspects of managing migraines effectively.

Homeopathic helpers

Belladonna: This remedy is indicated for migraines with intense throbbing pain that comes on suddenly. The person may experience sensitivity to light, noise, and jarring movements.

Nux vomica: Useful for migraines triggered by stress, overwork, or exposure to strong sensory stimuli. The person may have a headache with irritability, indigestion, and sensitivity to light and noise.

Gelsemium: Indicated for migraines that start at the back of the head and spread over the entire head. The person may experience heaviness, weakness, and dizziness along with the headache.

Iris versicolor: This remedy is suitable for migraines that involve intense, burning pain, usually on one side of the head. The person may experience nausea, vomiting, and a bitter taste in the mouth.

Sanguinaria canadensis: Useful for migraines that begin in the back of the head or neck and spread to the forehead or right eye. The person may experience throbbing or pulsating pain, along with nausea and vomiting.

MORNING SICKNESS

Morning sickness refers to nausea and vomiting that occurs during pregnancy, typically in the early stages. The exact cause of morning sickness is not fully understood, but it is believed to be related to hormonal changes and the increased sensitivity of the gastrointestinal system during pregnancy.

The choice of homeopathic remedy should be based on individual symptoms, the specific context of the morning sickness, and the person's overall health so it's advisable to consult with a qualified homeopath or healthcare professional for a proper evaluation. Additionally, maintaining good hydration, eating small, frequent meals, avoiding triggers, and getting plenty of rest can complement homeopathic treatment for morning sickness.

Homeopathic helpers

Nux vomica: This remedy is often indicated for morning sickness with nausea, retching, and a sensation of heaviness in the stomach. The person may feel irritable and have an aversion to odours and certain foods.

Ipecacuanha: It is suitable for morning sickness with persistent nausea and vomiting. The person may experience an excessive amount of saliva, but the vomiting does not provide relief.

Sepia: This remedy is used for morning sickness accompanied by a feeling of emptiness or faintness in the stomach. The person may have a lack of appetite, aversion to food, and feel exhausted.

Colchicum: It is indicated for morning sickness with extreme sensitivity to odours, which can trigger nausea and vomiting. The person may feel better with cold applications and may have a distaste for certain foods.

Pulsatilla: This remedy is helpful for morning sickness with mild nausea that worsens with certain foods. The person may have a changeable appetite, craving for rich or fatty foods, and feel better with fresh air.

PMS

Premenstrual syndrome (PMS) is a chronic condition refers to a collection of physical, emotional, and behavioural symptoms that occur in the days or weeks before menstruation. Common symptoms include mood swings, irritability, bloating, breast tenderness, fatigue, and food cravings. While PMS is a natural part of the menstrual cycle, severe or disruptive symptoms can significantly impact a woman's quality of life. Homeopathy offers natural remedies that can help alleviate PMS symptoms and restore balance. Additionally, lifestyle modifications such as regular exercise, a balanced diet, stress management, and getting enough rest can also help to managing PMS effectively.

Homeopathic helpers

Pulsatilla: This remedy is often indicated for women who experience mood swings, weepiness, and emotional sensitivity before their periods. They may have a strong desire for comfort and reassurance, and symptoms can improve with fresh air and gentle exercise.

Sepia: Useful for women with PMS who experience irritability, anger, and indifference towards loved ones. They may also have physical symptoms like hot flashes, fatigue, and a dragging sensation in the pelvis.

Natrum muriaticum: Indicated for women who become withdrawn and experience sadness, weepiness, and feelings of isolation during PMS. They may have a strong craving for salty foods and can be emotionally sensitive.

Lachesis: This remedy is suitable for women who experience intense irritability, jealousy, and mood swings during PMS. They may have physical symptoms such as hot flashes and headaches, and symptoms may worsen before or during periods.

Calcarea carbonica: Useful for women who experience fatigue, bloating, and weight gain before their periods. They may feel overwhelmed by responsibilities and have a craving for sweets and eggs.

Kirsty's story

Kirsty turned to homeopathy to help her with a severe case of premenstrual dysphoric disorder (PMDD)

I have suffered with Premenstrual Tension (PMT) for most of my adult life, but after my first child was born in 2003 my symptoms worsened considerably. Every month in the lead up to my period, I would experience the most overwhelming anger and depression. I would be going along with my day and then out of nowhere, it would feel like a piece of lead had dropped on me.

Everything was cloaked in despair

The depression was so severe that it got to the point where I couldn't function normally. I could be in bed for up to a week at a time, unable to go out or speak to anyone outside my family. I couldn't collect my son from school, prepare meals or take care of the running of the home. Everything was cloaked in despair, darkness and guilt. It was totally debilitating and I felt utterly hopeless. I didn't know where to turn.

Even more upsetting was the terrible and irrational rage I felt towards myself and my partner. It was so destructive. I don't know what I would have done if he hadn't been so strong, supportive and understanding.

In 2012, I was referred to a specialist clinic and diagnosed with PMDD. The only treatment they could offer was the contraceptive pill or an antidepressant, which I wasn't comfortable being on. I also tried beta blockers, but there was little improvement with any of these medications.

It transformed my life

I have always used homeopathy to treat minor ailments and illnesses, so I know about its ability to heal without side-effects. But I hadn't considered it as a treatment option for my PMDD as it seemed so unmanageable and overwhelming.

Eventually, in March 2022, my aunt persuaded me to visit see Dr Willocks at Coatbridge Homeopathy.

Lachesis was prescribed and within the first month, I started to feel an improvement. To say homeopathy has transformed my life would not be an overstatement.

For the first time in decades, I have little or no symptoms of PMDD-related rage and depression. My stress response has settled and I am noticeably calmer in situations that I would once have been unable to cope with.

My long-suffering partner—and my wonderfully understanding children—have all been amazed by the huge change in me. My whole family has benefited from the positive effects of this miraculous treatment."

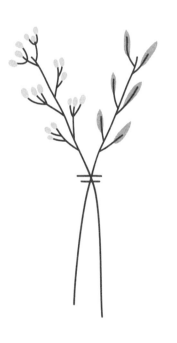

PSORIASIS

Psoriasis is a chronic condition that may require a combination of treatments, including homeopathy, topical medications, lifestyle modifications, and sometimes systemic medications, depending on the severity of the condition. If you have psoriasis, it's essential to work with a qualified healthcare professional, such as a dermatologist or a homeopath to develop a comprehensive treatment plan that addresses your specific needs.

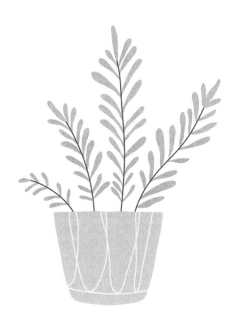

Homeopathic helpers

Graphites: This remedy is often used for psoriasis with thick, rough, and cracked skin. It can help alleviate itching and scaling and is especially useful when the condition worsens in cold weather.

Arsenicum album: When there are burning, itching, and restlessness associated with psoriasis, Arsenicum album may be considered. It can also address anxiety and restlessness.

Sulphur: This remedy is commonly used for psoriasis with intense itching, burning, and redness. It can be beneficial when the skin is dry and rough, and symptoms worsen with warmth.

Rhus toxicodendron: When psoriasis improves with movement and worsens with rest, Rhus toxicodendron may be helpful. It can address symptoms of itching, burning, and swelling.

Mezereum: This remedy is often used for psoriasis with thick, crusty, and oozing eruptions. It can assist in relieving itching and pain associated with the skin lesions.

SHINGLES

Also known as herpes zoster, this viral infection is caused by the varicella-zoster virus, the same virus that causes chickenpox. After a person recovers from chickenpox, the virus remains dormant in the nerve cells. However, it can reactivate later in life, leading to the development of shingles. The main symptom of shingles is a painful rash that typically occurs in a band or stripe on one side of the body.

Homeopathic remedies should be used under professional guidance to ensure proper dosing and monitoring of progress. Additionally, you should seek medical attention for shingles to prevent complications and receive appropriate medical care alongside homeopathic treatment.

Homeopathic helpers

Rhus tox: This remedy is often indicated for shingles with intense itching, burning, and restlessness. It can also help reduce inflammation and promote healing of the rash.

Mezereum: When the shingles rash is accompanied by intense neuralgic pain and burning, Mezereum may be considered. It can assist in relieving the pain and reducing the severity of the rash.

Apis mellifica: This remedy is commonly used for shingles with a blistering rash that is red, swollen, and accompanied by stinging and burning pain. It can help reduce inflammation and provide relief from pain and discomfort.

Ranunculus bulbosus: When the shingles rash is characterized by intense, neuralgic pain that is worse with touch or movement, Ranunculus bulbosus may be helpful. It can alleviate the pain and promote healing.

Arsenicum album: This remedy is often indicated when the shingles rash is accompanied by burning pain that is relieved by warm applications. It can also address restlessness and anxiety associated with shingles.

SPRAINS AND STRAINS

Homeopathy can provide supportive care in cases of sprains and strains, helping to reduce pain, inflammation, and promote healing. It's important to note that for severe injuries or fractures, immediate medical attention is necessary. However, for mild to moderate sprains and strains, homeopathy can work wonders. Additionally, applying cold compresses, resting the affected area, and using supportive measures like compression and elevation can complement treatment.

Homeopathic helpers

Arnica: Arnica is a well-known remedy for injuries, including sprains and strains. It can help reduce swelling, bruising, and alleviate pain. Arnica can be used topically as a cream or gel and taken orally in pellet form.

Ruta graveolens: It is indicated for injuries to tendons, ligaments, and cartilage. Ruta can help alleviate pain, stiffness, and promote the healing of strained or sprained tissues.

Rhus toxicodendron: This remedy is suitable for sprains or strains that worsen with initial movement but improve with continued motion. Rhus tox can help reduce stiffness, inflammation, and provide relief from pain.

Bryonia: It is indicated for sprains or strains that worsen with movement and are accompanied by intense pain and swelling. Bryonia can help reduce pain, swelling, and provide support during the healing process.

Calcarea phosphorica: This remedy is helpful for sprains or strains that involve slow healing or weak connective tissues. Calcarea phos can aid in tissue repair, strengthen ligaments and tendons, and promote recovery.

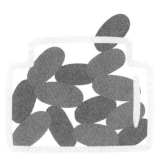

STRESS AND ANXIETY

Stress and anxiety have become increasingly common in our fast-paced lives. It can manifest as persistent worry, fear, nervousness, and physical symptoms such as rapid heartbeat, sweating, and difficulty concentrating. While it's essential to address the root causes and seek professional help when needed, homeopathy offers natural remedies that can help alleviate symptoms and promote emotional well-being. Lifestyle changes, stress management techniques, and seeking support from mental health professionals can also complement homeopathic treatment for stress and anxiety.

Homeopathic helpers

Aconitum napellus: This remedy is often indicated for acute panic attacks or sudden intense anxiety, especially after a shock or fright. You may experience a fear of death, restlessness, and a racing heart.

Arsenicum album: Useful for anxiety related to health concerns or fear of loss and insecurity. Good for perfectionist tendencies, feeling restless at night and experiencing a need for reassurance.

Ignatia amara: Indicated for grief, emotional shock, or sudden disappointment leading to anxiety and mood swings. You may suppress emotions and have a tendency to sigh or yawn frequently.

Gelsemium sempervirens: Helpful for anticipatory anxiety, stage fright, and performance anxiety. You may feel weak, tremble, and experience a sense of heaviness.

Lycopodium clavatum: Suitable for anxiety related to low self-esteem and fear of failure. Good for irritability, digestive issues and a desire for warm food.

Argentum nitricum: Indicated for anxiety associated with anticipation, such as before exams, public speaking, or important events. Helps strong craving for sweets and digestive issues.

Natrum muriaticum: Useful for chronic anxiety related to past grief or emotional trauma. It can help if you are sensitive to criticism and experience a fear of rejection.

SEASONAL AFFECTIVE DISORDER

Seasonal Affective Disorder (SAD) is a type of depression that typically occurs during certain seasons, most commonly in the fall and winter months when daylight hours are shorter. It is thought to be related to a lack of sunlight, which can disrupt the body's internal clock and affect mood-regulating chemicals in the brain. Symptoms of SAD may include feelings of sadness, fatigue, loss of interest in activities, changes in appetite, difficulty concentrating, and increased need for sleep. Homeopathy offers natural remedies that may help alleviate the symptoms of Seasonal Affective Disorder and support emotional well-being. In addition, light therapy, regular exercise, maintaining a healthy diet and lifestyle.

Homeopathic helpers

Natrum muriaticum: This remedy is often indicated for SAD with symptoms such as sadness, isolation, and withdrawal. The person may have an increased appetite for salty foods and feel worse in the mornings.

Aurum metallicum: Useful for SAD with feelings of hopelessness, sadness, and a loss of interest in life. The person may have suicidal thoughts and feel worse at night.

Pulsatilla: Indicated for SAD with symptoms such as weepiness, mood swings, and a desire for consolation. The person may crave comforting foods and feel better with fresh air and gentle exercise.

Ignatia amara: This remedy is suitable for SAD with symptoms of emotional sensitivity, mood swings, and a tendency to suppress emotions. The person may experience sudden outbursts of crying or laughter.

Lycopodium: Useful for SAD with symptoms of low self-esteem, irritability, and digestive issues. The person may have a fear of being alone and feel worse in the late afternoon and evening.

Remedy finder at a glance

While homeopathic remedies should be selected based on individualized symptoms, and consulting a qualified homeopath or healthcare professional is recommended for accurate diagnosis and treatment, below are some common ailments and the remedies that are traditionally used to treat them.

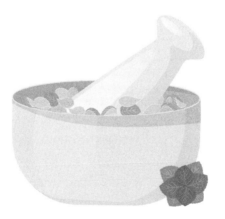

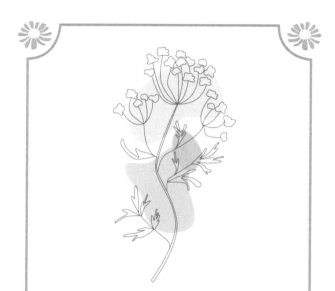

Acne: Belladonna, Hepar sulphuris, Kali bromatum, Pulsatilla

Allergies: Allium cepa, Euphrasia, Natrum muriaticum, Sabadilla

Anxiety: Argentum nitricum, Gelsemium, Ignatia amara, Lycopodium

Arthritis: Bryonia, Rhus toxicodendron, Colchicum, Ledum palustre

Asthma: Arsenicum album, Ipecacuanha, Natrum sulphuricum, Sambucus nigra

Bronchitis: Antimonium tartaricum, Bryonia, Phosphorus, Pulsatilla

Cold and flu: Aconite, Belladonna, Eupatorium perfoliatum, Nux vomica

Constipation: Bryonia, Nux vomica, Opium, Sepia

Cough: Drosera, Hepar sulphuris, Spongia tosta, Sticta pulmonaria

Depression: Aurum metallicum, Ignatia amara, Natrum sulphuricum, Pulsatilla

Diarrhoea: Arsenicum album, Podophyllum, Pulsatilla, Veratrum album

Earache: Belladonna, Chamomilla, Pulsatilla, Silicea

Eczema: Arsenicum album, Graphites, Sulphur, Mezereum

Fatigue: China officinalis, Kali phosphoricum, Nux vomica, Phosphoricum acidum

Headache: Belladonna, Bryonia, Gelsemium, Natrum muriaticum

Haemorrhoids: Aesculus hippocastanum, Hamamelis, Nux vomica, Sulphur

Insomnia: Coffea cruda, Nux vomica, Passiflora incarnata, Lycopodium

Menstrual Problems: Pulsatilla, Sepia, Lachesis, Sabina

Migraine: Belladonna, Iris versicolor, Natrum muriaticum, Sanguinaria

Nausea: Nux vomica, Ipecacuanha, Colchicum, Tabacum

Osteoporosis: Calcarea carbonica, Silicea, Symphytum, Ruta graveolens

PMS (Premenstrual Syndrome): Lachesis, Natrum muriaticum, Pulsatilla, Sepia

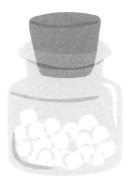

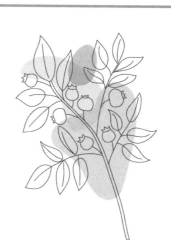

Psoriasis: Arsenicum album, Graphites, Sulphur, Mezereum
Sinusitis: Kali bichromicum, Pulsatilla, Silicea, Hydrastis
Sore Throat: Belladonna, Mercurius solubilis, Lachesis, Phytolacca
Stress: Argentum nitricum, Ignatia amara, Natrum muriaticum, Arsenicum album
Sunburn: Cantharis, Belladonna, Apis mellifica, Urtica urens

Teething Problems: Chamomilla, Belladonna, Calcarea carbonica, Coffea cruda

Tonsillitis: Belladonna, Mercurius solubilis, Lachesis, Phytolacca

Urinary Tract Infection (UTI): Cantharis, Apis mellifica, Staphysagria, Pulsatilla

Varicose Veins: Hamamelis, Pulsatilla, Calcarea fluorica, Lycopodium

Vertigo: Cocculus indicus, Conium maculatum, Bryonia, Gelsemium

Warts: Thuja occidentalis, Causticum, Antimonium crudum, Dulcamara

ACKNOWLEDGMENTS

I could not have written this book without the superb help and guidance from the dedicated team at Homeopathy UK, which is the UK's leading charity for the promotion of homeopathy. The charity's mission is for everyone to understand the value of homeopathy and be able to access high-quality treatment from registered healthcare professionals. Homeopathy UK runs a network of free charitable clinics around the UK, provides information such as an online 'Find a Homeopath' tool and publishes a magazine—*Health & Homeopathy*—three times a year. The charity also provides grants to specialist clinics supporting vulnerable groups such as military veterans and domestic abuse victims. For more information, visit www.homeopathy-uk.org.

FOR REFERENCE

Information for the public

Homeopathy UK—www.homeopathy-uk.org

UK registering bodies

The Faculty of Homeopathy—https://www.facultyofhomeopathy.org/
The Society of Homeopaths—https://homeopathy-soh.org/
The Alliance of Registered Homeopaths—Alliance of Registered Homeopaths—https://www.a-r-h.org

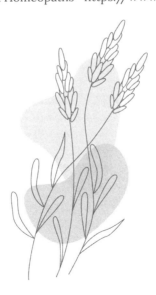

Pharmacies

Helios—https://www.helios.co.uk/
Ainsworths—https://www.ainsworths.com/
Nelsons—https://www.nelsonspharmacy.com/

Research

Homeopathic Research Institute—https://www.
hri-research.org/

Education

https://www.findahomeopath.org/courses

Animals

Whole Health Agriculture—https://wholehealthag.
org/
Homeopathy at Wellie Level—https://www.hawl.
co.uk/
British Association of Homeopathic Vets—https://
bahvs.net/